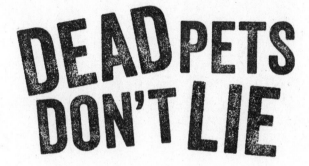

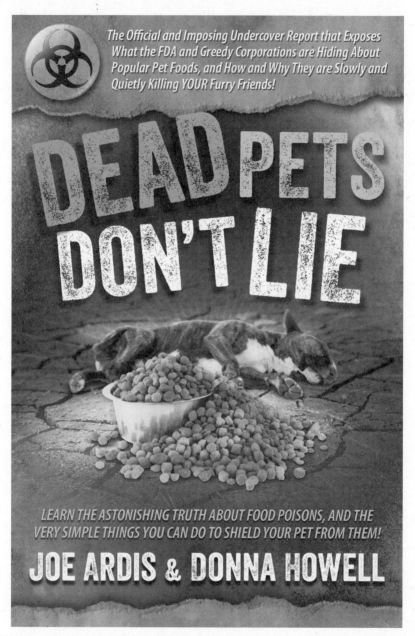

The Official and Imposing Undercover Report that Exposes What the FDA and Greedy Corporations are Hiding About Popular Pet Foods, and How and Why They are Slowly and Quietly Killing YOUR Furry Friends!

DEAD PETS DON'T LIE

LEARN THE ASTONISHING TRUTH ABOUT FOOD POISONS, AND THE VERY SIMPLE THINGS YOU CAN DO TO SHIELD YOUR PET FROM THEM!

JOE ARDIS & DONNA HOWELL

DEFENDER PUBLISHING

CRANE, MO 65633

DEAD PETS DON'T LIE

The Official and Imposing Undercover Report That Exposes What the FDA and Greedy Corporations Are Hiding about Popular Pet Foods, and How and Why They Are Slowly and Quietly Killing YOUR Furry Friends! THE ASTONISHING TRUTH AND THE VERY SIMPLE THINGS YOU CAN DO TO SHEILD YOUR PETS FROM FOOD POISONS THAT ARE KEEPING THEM FROM HAPPIER, HEALTHIER, LONGER LIVES!

©2015 by Joe Ardis and Donna Howell.

All rights reserved. Published 2015.

Printed in the United States of America.

ISBN 13: 978-0-9964095-2-0

A CIP catalog record of this book is available from the Library of Congress.

Cover illustration and design by Jeffrey Mardis.

Author cover photography by Angelina Keepper.

Contents

Foreword

By Thomas Horn,
CEO of Defender Publishing, SkyWatch TV,
and Whispering Ponies Ranch

Because my work is generally viewed by society as the public's voice of concern, responding to alarming human science and technology, very few actually know that I have a great wealth of concern *also* for the proper treatment of animals.

Although it's accurate to say that I have always cared about the animal kingdom, my love for animals increased a couple decades ago as a result of my experience as an executive on the board of Camp and Conference Ministries on the West Coast. The CCM were overseers of four camping and retreat facilities in the state of Oregon, one of which had fallen into great disrepair. Wishing to see this absolutely beautiful land restored to its potential, I agreed to move there for a few years to assist with reconstruction. This camp was located between two crater lakes, in what you might call a "wilderness" location, and over the years as the construction improved the facility, I observed many crowds flocking to this place for their own personal restoration and study. We saw to the needs of many groups, including religious, nonreligious, women's, men's, teenage youth, children's, outdoor schools, Future Farmers of America, Girl Scouts, Boy Scouts, and many more. By the time we were fully operational and had achieved accreditation in the American Camping Association as well as financial backing from the Murdock Foundation and Ford Family Foundation, it was nearly impossible to book a week at our site.

As the crowds flocked in to "get away from it all," creating a mounting list of fond memories and people interactions I would relish for years to come, one particular group stood out above the rest and made a profound impression on me—for life. They were known as the "Royal Family Kids Camp."

Kids from troubled backgrounds (or whose parents had passed away) who had ended up as wards of the state gathered once per year at our camp. Most often, these children had been emotionally, physically, or psychologically damaged during the past, and they had lost their trust in people. Many of them were completely shut down socially, which presented a major problem in their rehabilitation. As a result of this unusual situation, each child was assigned to a specific "trustee," and most of the communication happened through that one individual. Even our retreat staff was strictly instructed not to speak to these kids unless they spoke to one of us first (in which case we were to be as polite and kind as possible, but we were to keep communication to a minimum). The bond between each child and his or her trustee was a critical alliance that could not be placed at risk during this sensitive time in the child's life.

People, as these children had sadly learned, could hurt you.

But in addition to the trustees, this group had utilized interaction with *animals* to pull some of these young ones out of the despair they had been in for so long. I was amazed that it hadn't occurred to me before of the importance of human/animal interaction in a therapeutic setting. It's astonishing how a small puppy or a horse can connect with a human in ways other humans never will.

These children knew on an innate and instinctive level that these animals had no abusive agenda. That puppy, kitten, or pony was not waiting for a child to let his or her guard down to gain a manipulative edge and turn on the young person later. No calm and tender creature like those I witnessed would ever turn on the child in the way humans had. These small kids may not have been able to put into words why they reached out with open trust toward a furry little companion, but they did so nonetheless, and with complete abandon of all other cares.

In that moment, that one moment shared between a pet companion and a child, there was no more hurt or suffering or fear. For the duration of their connection, the only emotion observable from the outside was joy and camaraderie.

The way this program was used to help the children reintegrate into society—developing trust first with an animal and then with a human—led to these injured lives becoming whole again. And *that* healing process, of all the things I saw during my days with the CCM, meant the very most.

I had always valued animals, but *now* I had come to understand a higher purpose for them. And the success stories were not limited to trained therapy animals. The experience of watching the children in the Royal Family Kids Camp opened my eyes to see everywhere around me the bond between mankind and our companions. My awareness of humanity's need for these soft, gentle creatures heightened with such a speed that I began to recognize the importance of this connection everywhere in daily life, on TV, in public, in the news... All around me, the truth was evident: Animals can connect with humanity in ways humanity fails.

They are a gift to us, a treasure...an extreme value.

And, as such, they should be *treated* as if they are the valuable, treasured gifts that they are.

I was not completely unaware of the red flags in the pet food industry before Joe Ardis and Donna Howell approached me with the disturbing facts contained in this book. I had, of course, heard that what the majority of people are feeding their animals was less than ideal. But the *measure* to which the industry has knowingly participated in providing the most nutritionally void, dangerous "foods" to pet owners—and the *lengths* at which they will travel to keep their detestable food practices a secret while masquerading their products as "healthy" with clever advertising schemes and suspect endorsements... All that was new information, and I found it shocking.

The information you will read in this book is well researched, well documented, relevant to all pet owners, and the most cutting-edge whistle-blower within its genre.

For the sincere pet owners: Words cannot express how much you need to read this book and learn from its revelations. In the evenings, since I have read it personally, I now rest easier knowing that I no longer fall prey to the deceit, and that the diet my loyal guard dog receives is an incredible improvement as a result of Joe Ardis and Donna Howell's work. I give it my highest level of recommendation.

Our pets are an invaluable gift to us. Cherish them. Feed them well.

And read this book.

Introduction

Killing Your Pet

*I care not for a man's religion whose dog
and cat are not the better for it.*
—ABRAHAM LINCOLN[1]

So, you finally took the plunge and got yourself a pet. Maybe your decision was the result of several years of diligent planning and obsessive breed research. Perhaps your local pet store window showcased a kitten with all the spots in all the right places and you just couldn't pass it up. Perhaps that nice lady down the street in the cool RV with dangly wind chimes had a fresh litter of fur balls in a cardboard box with a "free" sign and one particularly adorable face in the mix. Or, possibly you've had Fido for years and can't imagine your life without that amazing, loyal hound dog. Whatever the original reason for adding a pet to your home, you couldn't help yourself, and we don't blame you.

By choosing to share your life with a trustworthy companion, you've entered a demographic category shared by millions. We've all heard that endearing proverbial phrase about dogs being man's best friends, and many times the phrase has been adjusted to suit each person's own beloved pet species. Entering pet ownership is, as you well know, not unique. According to the *2012 U.S. Pet Ownership & Demographics Sourcebook*, more than 70 percent of American households own dogs, cats, birds, or horses as pets. A great majority of the remaining less than 30 percent of American households have a pet from within the secondary categories such as rodents and reptiles.[2] Animals have an undeniably magnetic pull on the lion's share of humans (you know, that *other* hairy species occupying the planet). We love to pat the head of that friend on our lap; we can't wait to scratch behind the ears of the protector that will bark at night-time intruders; we appreciate listening to the comforting sound of the ever-present purring of that kitty cat on the windowsill; and we can't keep from uttering that "aww" of admiration when we see the newborn puffball on shaky legs for the first time, mewing or whimpering for its four-legged mama's milk. This animal shows concern with no strings attached, picks up on our times of emotional need, and finds ways of "listening" to our troubles without judgment.

In return, we show them great affection, provide them comfy homes, make them one of the family, and give them only the best…

Or *do* we?

Looking at it another way: Humans have adopted many species of animals out of their natural habitats over time and domesticated them to live by our standards and rules. Many of us expect them to understand and obey our human languages and respond immediately to our complicated explanations regarding their undesirable behaviors while their own psychological needs as non-humans are not being met. We buy them squeaky toys and wonder why they're not happy. Yet, without the psychological fulfillment of their needs, our pets go crazy and spin in circles when we want to sit and relax. Then, every day, tens of thousands of Americans unknowingly provide pets with poison in their feeding dishes that shortens their lives and delivers their bodies to cancerous, tumor-inducing health conditions and, often, slow and painful deaths. It's quite a puzzling piece of poetry, this. But don't take *our* word for it; the research in this book cites international pet food authorities, well-respected and groundbreaking news releases, Freedom of Information (FOI) documents, esteemed animal rights associations, certified and licensed pet care physicians, experts in biology, professionals in holistic pet care, and many other reliable sources within the scientific community, as well as some personal interviews with respected individuals within their industry of practice.

Humans are a funny species. We are by far the most intelligent beings on planet earth; still, millions of people worldwide fall victim to clever media campaigns and propaganda within the commercial industry, investing time, money, and resources in dishonest claims. Intelligence, as we imagine everyone already knows, is not the same as wisdom or perception. As the great Italian composer Gian Carlo Menotti once said, "A man only becomes wise when he begins to calculate the approximate depth of his ignorance."[3] And ignorance is certainly not the same as stupidity. Ignorance is simply the lack of information or knowledge, and it's certainly not something to be ashamed of, until it is intentionally embraced as a result of the fear of truth or responsibility to act once truth is obtained: a mistake that humanity has all too often made.

We've probably all seen some variant of the following commercial: Fade in on a dog running in slow-motion, with a shining coat and perfect teeth, frolicking through the grass in the back yard playing Frisbee with his owner. The sun is bright; the owner is trim and healthy, and wears spotless clothing. As energetic playtime commences, suggesting to the viewer a positive atmosphere ripe with exercise and fitness, some charming voiceover begins to talk about the well being of man's best friend and the bond between humans and animals (sometimes conveying a touchy back story). Then the narrative may turn toward discussing the harmful ingredients of some competing dog food and why, if *you* care about your pet, you'll only feed him the best. Persuasion drops just before the end of the footage in corny sayings that resonate subtleties likened to, "For a friendship this great, owners only give their *best* friends the *best*." (Note that this is not a real commercial catchphrase that we know of, but it might as well be.) Then, as heaping portions of food—more than any canine really requires in order to thrive—are poured into the dish, the happy tail-wagger devours it without hesitation, suggesting amongst so many other things that the dog finds the food appetizing. The commercial-brand bag appears off to the side of the screen, listing convincing facts about the food, usually pertaining to all the vitamins or protein your pet will receive as a benefit of choosing this brand. Almost invariably, the imagery and touchy-feely representation of the overall commercial experience leads viewers to believe *this* dog food is healthier than all the others, and if *their* dog is special enough to them, if *their* dog is "like family" (oh-so-many commercials drop that little zinger), then the viewer will do the caring thing, the "only what's best" thing, and drive straight to the store for this brand of chow. Somewhere in the midst of this order, a man in a lab coat appears with a line about how this particular food is "recommended by vets"—adding reassurance of nutritional value. The pitch is bought, hook, line, and sinker, by the majority. Certainly not everyone is going to buy into whatever commercials advertise, but with the real information and facts obscured from everyday media when it comes to pet foods, a lot of people are consistently fooled by cunning advertisements. As a sad addition, many paid employees at pet stores or commercial department stores unintentionally misinform the public by referring to handy five-point charts or memorized fact sheets, but they are only repeating what they have been told by the biased food companies, themselves.

Let's just get this out of the way: If people are willing to believe the clever phraseology in pet food commercials or sales pitches, then they should save a lot of time, money, and grief by simply giving their pet a bowl full of discarded yellow grass from the neighbor's lawn mower bag. It would be healthier, anyway. Millions of Americans are unknowingly killing their beloved pets every day by feeding them foods riddled with toxic, foreign, unnatural, kidney-damaging, heart-disease-promoting, and cancer-creating foods that are linked to blood disease, still births, premature deaths, and more health conditions than we can list in this quick introduction. And this is all aside from the plethora of terrible medical interventions for pet health concerns. Issues such as flea problems, skin conditions, allergies, shedding, and weight management, as well as countless other maladies, are not only treated with harsh chemicals (that only *appear* to work, while, in reality, the lethal chemicals take forever to leave your pet's body and the problem comes back full swing), but they also cause distressing side effects that require more medication—thus beginning the vicious cycle of constant, cascading veterinarian or pharmaceutical intervention. "Professionals," including local vets, are *sometimes* the least and last informed of how these medications are completely ineffective and incredibly harmful to your pet, and *sometimes*, the professionals are part of the problem, because they work to perpetuate extreme treatments for a list of reasons we will visit in more depth later.

You may be thinking: *Is this real? Don't we live in the great USA? How can the FDA be allowing the poisoning of our pets, assuming it's true? Aren't there laws ensuring safe pet food ingredients and medications? How is it possible that shoppers are fooled every day? How can this be happening? Wouldn't mega chain stores be dealing with lawsuits if this really is taking place?*

There may be readers who think this book surely isn't speaking to *them*, of all people, because *they* get "Fill-In-the-Blank" healthy pet food brand, so *they* must be in the clear. If that is you, then, yes, we are also talking to you. You are not any more immune to the secrecy of commercialization than anyone else in the great US of A. It's all about money and business, and the health and longevity of your pet is the least of our government's concern.

Wouldn't thousands of pets be dying as a result of this?
Yes, they would be, and they are.
Yeah, but I shop at Walmart, and Walmart would never…
Yes it would, it does, and it will.
But the government would never allow…
Yes they would, they do, and they will.

Many feed their pets deadly food or administer dangerous medicine because they don't have the time or the interest in researching the shocking truth about what the food and drug companies are hiding, but the very fact that you purchased this book shows that you have an increased concern in providing only the best nutrition for your pet. Congratulations on taking the first step toward *wisdom*, and toward giving *your* "best friend" the "best."

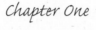

Chapter One

The Big Commercial Lie

If you tell a big enough lie and tell it
frequently enough, it will be believed.
—ADOLF HITLER[4]

With more than eighty-three million dogs and more than ninety-six million cats living in US homes today,[5] it comes as no surprise that Americans will spend over $21 billion ($31.3 billion, adjusted for inflation since 1996) on pet food this year,[6] and that number is only growing. According to *CBS News Money Watch* last March:

> Americans spent an all-time high of $55.7 billion on their pets in the last year and spending will creep close to $60 billion this year [2014], an industry spokesman said Thursday.
>
> Pets across America live like little humans these days—and as long as people treat them that way, pet spending should keep climbing, said Bob Vetere, the

president and CEO of the American Pet Products Association. Overall pet spending has not dipped since record-keeping started, according to APPA [American Pet Products Association], based in Greenwich, Connecticut.

The biggest part of spending in 2013—$21.57 billion—went for food—a lot of it more expensive, *healthier* grub, Vetere told buyers and exhibitors at the Global Pet Expo in Orlando, Florida. The not-for-profit trade association has been tracking industry figures since 1996, when total pet spending was just $21 billion. Adjusted for inflation, that's $31.3 billion.[7]

The size and scope of pet food options, especially those that claim to offer the most nutrition, is staggering. Trying to decipher nutritional labels or wade through all the rhetoric sales people are pitching as to why *their* brand of pet food is the best value on the market, and how it is nutritionally balanced to meet all of the needs of your pet, can be extremely challenging. Unfortunately, many of the foods offered by mega-chain stores are pumped full of kidney-damaging scent enhancers that entice pets to eat vigorously so their owners assume their pets really like that particular food. Dyes make the food appear to have a variety of different components, when in fact, there are not. Devastatingly dangerous preservatives ensure an unnaturally long shelf life, so that the manufacturers have a larger window of time in which to sell the food and improve their bottom line.

And this is just the tip of the iceberg.

Sadly, many of these foods are sold to mass consumers

who believe the manufacturers' claims of being committed to the health and longevity of our precious animals, when in fact, the products they're creating have been linked to pet cancer and hair loss; heart, kidney, and liver failure; still births; blood disorders; and premature death—just to name a few. As many have heard on television ads, the food choices you make for your pet can affect their behavior as well (one of the few truthful statements these commercials make), which exacerbates the frustration many owners face when choosing a brand, since many labels also claim to provide the ingredients that will promote a "happy" pet, and then fail to deliver.

Understanding the Lie

Medical studies have illustrated that when we feed our children heavy loads of sugar, they can become depressed, anxious, hyper, emotionally angry, and less social…and the list goes on and on. Sugar is just one ingredient we can link to dozens of behavioral challenges regarding our children. It's possible you've heard that this idea about sugar is all an old wives' tale. On one hand, that's true. Many studies throughout the last several decades show that sugar doesn't make kids hyper or moody. On the other hand, excess sugar is terrible for the body, *and* for moods.

How can both angles be true?

In order to understand the lie in animal food commercialization, let's quickly visit one erroneous factor in our understanding of sugar.

Of course, there have been uncountable studies debunking the myth that a lollipop will induce a child to hyperactivity, but we aren't talking about an occasional lollipop, and we aren't just addressing hyperactivity. Exorbitant amounts of sugar can affect the health and moods of both children and adults. When an adult experiences mood swings after eating an entire cheesecake in one sitting, because there is no direct parent who must assume responsibility or deal with the reaction, many people fail to make the connection, writing off the grown-up meltdown to having "a bad day." When a child is the center of focus, throwing a tantrum in the toy aisle after a bowl of Frosted Flakes, confused parents unite in a worldwide and historical "the-sugar-made-them-do-it" misconception. It's far more complicated than that.

Putting it simply, sugar alone generally has no effect on a person's mood. A Google search on "the effects of sugar on children's behavior" indicates that this myth of hyperactivity or mood swings as a direct result of sugar intake has been debunked by hundreds of studies, most within the last fifteen years. As *WebMD* reported in 1999:

In the past 10 years, several studies have examined the effects of sugar on children's behavior. Here are the aspects of the studies that make them credible:

- Known quantities of sugar in the diets were studied.
- The studies compared the effects of sugar with those of a placebo (a substance without any active ingredients).

- The children, parents and researchers involved in the studies never knew which children were given which diets (this is known as a "double-blind" study and helps to prevent unconscious biases from affecting the results).
- An analysis of the results of all these studies was published in the November 22, 1995 issue of the *Journal of the American Medical Association.* The researchers' conclusions? Sugar in the diet *did not* affect the children's behavior.[8]

But how can this be, when surely everyone knows that sugar makes kids bounce off the walls and then "crash" into depression? It's common knowledge, right? So, is the science wrong on this one? Or is the cultural association to an assumption made by the Shannon Clinic in 1922 so imprinted on our minds that we're imagining the link?

Both camps are correct: Sugar generally has no effect on moods, but observing mood swings after sugar is very real. The confusion? It's not what sugar does to the mood, it's what sugar does to a person's glucose balance. A sudden and heavy intake of sugar causes peaks and dips in the amount of glucose in the blood, causing "fatigue, irritability, dizziness, insomnia, excessive sweating (especially at night), poor concentration and forgetfulness, excessive thirst, depression and crying spells, digestive disturbances and blurred vision."[9] A disruption of blood glucose levels can easily produce mood swings in people of all ages.

Let's use a commercial regarding sugar as an example: If

a candy company were to create a candy bar containing the same sugar as any other candy company and then release a promotional video on their website stating that the sugar *they* used would not cause hyperactivity in a child, it could be considered as technically true, because standard sugar doesn't cause hyperactivity in a child. What the candy company wouldn't be telling you is that the sugar *they* used (meaning the standard sugar every other candy company is using) is responsible for upsetting the balance of blood glucose in a child, which can cause hyperactivity followed by "crashing."

So, essentially, in a world where people are unwilling to research the claims of an ad about candy bars, a company could release a product it claims to be "healthier" than the rest, and millions would buy the product. The reason a *candy* company couldn't get by with that specific claim is because the world would see it on television, do a double take, realize on an innate level that it goes against everything they know, and be all over it with research and response. As soon they discovered the deception, people all over the place would be blogging about the terrible, lying company and the harmful ingredients it uses. This would be marketing suicide. The "whole truth" is what people want, and when they are scammed, they react. Everyone already knows that sugar is very harmful to the human body in high and frequent doses, so no candy company will attempt to pull the wool over the nation's eyes with this one merely because of the public's preexisting awareness of sugar's harmful properties.

And yet...when pet food companies do the exact same thing, claiming that their foods are packed with wonderful, protein-filled ingredients, vitamins, and vegetables, and portray healthy dogs bounding through meadows in the sunshine, most people won't dig deep enough to expose the outrageous lie that there is more about these pet foods than the commercials are telling everyone.

Why not?

Three reasons:

1) *People* don't eat pet food, so *people* don't research pet foods the way they would human food.

2) People don't have previously existing, imprinted opinions about the effects of harmful pet food ingredients (as they have about sugar's effects on human behavior, like the example above).

3) Pets don't speak human languages, so they can't communicate to us that something in their food is making them sick. Thus, we fail to be flagged to negative physical symptoms (and behavioral symptoms) the way we are when our sugar-crashing children consume exorbitant amounts of "special" candy bars that promised to hold special, healthier properties.

The pet industry *can* fool people into buying dangerous pet food, so they *do*. When compared to common and openly repeated facts about sugar's effect on the human body that society constantly reminds us of from birth and beyond, pet food facts are scarce and conflicting. The number of people who study pet food ingredients versus those who study human food ingredients is incomparable.

Animals can't communicate like us. They can't tell us that their belly hurts or that the slow poisoning from what's going into their dishes is diligently killing them. They can't bring us up to speed on their dietary observations. We don't often know what our pets are thinking or feeling. When they throw little behavioral tantrums or their health starts to fail, instead of saying that "sugar made them do it" or that their diet is responsible, we chalk it up to "bad training," "poor breeding," or the fact that "dogs/cats just don't live that long."

And consider the frequency of feedings: If children are affected by something going on in their body and they communicate it with "I want that toy!" followed by incessant weeping, at the very least, a parent can connect the dots between the child's behavior and the birthday cake he or she ate an hour beforehand, because *cake is not the only food item the child is eating*. If a child were to be given birthday cake two or three times daily as the only nutrition source for a prolonged period of time, nobody in his right mind would question the cause of the child's mood swings. Concern over behavioral problems would surely be second to immediate intervention for parental negligence. The child would likely be obese and develop early diabetes, and the chances that he would eventually fuel a potential cancer growth are much, *much* higher. "Early death" and severe health problems occurring within the body of a human fed nothing but birthday cake for years on end is a no-brainer.

People usually feed their pets the same food two or three times daily—and that's typically all they are given. (This is not necessarily a bad thing, assuming the food is healthy in the first place, although many veterinarians *do* recommend changing pet diets every few weeks [see "Interview with a Holistic Veterinarian"].) When the food source is toxic, a pet, much like a child, will become uncomfortable, sick, and maybe even cranky. Then, when that pet develops cancer, starts having an itchy coat, develops droopy eyelids, doesn't catch on to proper training, shows aggression, or demonstrates irrational mood swings, people assume the problem has originated in the pet.

If you are a concerned, loving parent, you are *not* going to feed your child birthday cake several times a day for years, because you care about him (or her), and want him to live long and thrive. You don't want him to become ill and possibly face premature death. You care about him, and not just because you get to cuddle him and watch him grow (although that's a huge contributing factor), but because it is your responsibility as a sensible and reliable parent to bring up your child in the most humane and painless way, because he is a living, breathing entity who relies on your care.

Why should paying attention to what we feed our pets be any different?

Our Responsibility as the Dominating Species

In North America, the FDA has already put a stop to many harmful ingredients and food practices as they pertain to *human consumption*. Nobody can accurately claim that the FDA has already arrived at a perfected system wherein everything a human consumes is perfectly safe—certainly not. But where people are concerned, a great effort has been made by the regulatory entities that we rely upon to ensure that what we put into our bodies meets a certain standard of health. The same cannot *at all* be said about what goes into our pets' food.

And what does that say about our society, when ingredients proven to cause cancer, illness, premature death, and terrible health side effects in humans have been approved for *animal consumption*? (More on FDA regulations in chapter 2.)

In the opinion of these authors, this shows that something is wrong with our culture's indicative mindset. It represents an attitude toward the care of animals that *simply is not what it should be*! Regardless of religious convictions, culture differences, lifestyle variations, and all other issues that contribute to the diversity of mankind as it relates to animal care, we share a responsibility as the dominating species to watch over the minority species.

Here in the states, we would never intentionally bring a human child into our home, feel the frustration of raising that child, decide the child is an improper match for our household, and then casually list him or her for sale on Craigslist like we do with pets that "just don't work out." We would never adopt a child from an agency and then put him or her in a fighting ring and watch as he or she battles it out in some sick, old-world, fight-to-the-death, gladiator-style entertainment routine like we do with pit bulls in modern-day, illegal fighting rings. We would not create baby mills or have baby backyard breeders placing tiny humans in terrible, substandard, health-threatening living conditions for the purpose of cranking out huge numbers of cute babies to sell like the puppy mills and backyard breeders do with canines.

As another example: We would not compromise the

genetic makeup of human children by selectively breeding them into the womb with narrower noses because it's cosmetically appealing to society, and then submit those same children to painful, "corrective" surgeries when their noses end up a little *too* narrow. But breeders do this very thing when they selectively breed forward the most wrinkly-faced Chinese shar-peis and bull dogs to create unnaturally wrinkly offspring because society think it looks cute and snuggly, only to turn around and put them under the scalpel for *wrinkle-reduction surgery* when their faces appear a little *too* wrinkly. (That's not to mention that the areas between the flaps of loose skin are bacterial breeding grounds, requiring additional maintenance that most owners don't keep up with and creating poor hygienic conditions for the dog.) Many admirers don't understand that these dogs were not meant by nature to have such an excess of skin covering their faces and sinuses, which can cause respiratory and sinus distress, airflow blockage and obscured vision, making even normal activity difficult. (Again, when this occurs, we have to correct what the breeding has done by subjecting them to painful surgeries.)

There are, of course, exceptions to the rule in our respect for humanity: from impulsive child adoptions that end too casually to psychopathic murderers who place their victims in insane, gladiator-like situations. And surely there are crazy scientists out there looking into how to breed people with vain specifications. However, the reaction of the human race around them speaks of an expectation—no, a *demand*—for better treatment and respect for human life. The outrage and protests that would ensue upon the unveiling of humankind's abuse under such circumstances would be intense and vigorous.

Using the pit bull fighting rings as a further example of this comparison: If someone were to adopt a human boy, keep him in a cage, poke at him, provoke him to anger, starve him to near death, and then release him to take out his aggression in a ring against another child, that person would likely go to prison for life and potentially face the death sentence if human life had been lost as a consequence. But Anthony Reddick—a thug who already faced two convictions of dog fighting—was *not* under a very effective and watchful eye from our police force as he continued to obtain, train, and release pit bulls in their bloody rings of death despite his criminal record. In February of 2014, he was arrested for setting a garage on fire to exterminate thirteen ferocious dogs—that he was responsible for training to be killers—ranging from two and a half months to five years old. (Note that many of the animals rescued or found in these types of situations, whose histories are associated with violent events such as barbaric fighting, end up being euthanized because they are deemed unadoptable.) Reddick's sentence? Three years in prison and a prohibition from owning animals for fifteen years.[10] Not only will he be reintegrated into free society within three years of his incarceration date, but by the year 2030, he will once again be allowed to own, and therefore *train*, animals. Because of his previous run-ins with the law and repeat offenses, these authors have no reason to believe that Reddick won't immediately run out and add more dogs' lives to the terrible, bloody body count.

Yet, the Anthony Reddick case is *small news* compared to

some of today's headlines. Few have heard of Reddick's crimes, but in turn, the media swarms around news of which Hollywood star has lost weight, which celebrity married whom, or what television show is popular. How can the matters of animal well-being be dismissed so easily from the media? Where is the outrage? Where is the public's interest? And why do the consequences of animal cruelty seem so irrelevant to society compared to the consequences of other crimes? Why does culture regard the treatment of animals with such a casual, dismissive approach?

Some believe that animals are God's creation, meant to live alongside us as companions. Others believe that they are a product of evolution and have come about in the same way that we humans have: as a result of a "big bang." Those who hold the former belief should respect animals because they *are* God's creation: put on this earth to share our world, comfort us, and befriend us in our never-ending striving toward righteousness—a side effect of which would be to appreciate and take care of everything God has entrusted to us. Those who associate with the latter belief owe animals respect simply because nature put them here via evolutionary means—in which case, who are we to decide what species of nature is of more importance than another? Does not equal means of creation via evolution produce equal rights to coexist, and, thus, *at least* close-to-equal concern for the welfare of all natural creation despite which species is more intelligent?

Regardless of the driving force behind a conviction to care for animals—be it religious or secular—these authors doubt that anyone could create a convincing argument for why mistreating or neglecting our animals should be a normative approach in this or any other wealthy nation with the resources to be actively involved in their welfare.

And yet, the FDA allowing our pets to consume harmful foods that have been deemed unfit for humans is only one reflection of the Western frame of mind. The fact that we tolerate the FDA allowing foods that would kill or create illnesses in animals, while refusing to allow those same practices in the business of human foods, says something about *us*. As humans, many don't value the rest of creation in the best way, given that we're the most dominant species. We can decide this priority for ourselves and yet subject the rest of creation to a lesser form of moral responsibility.

Imagine a species bigger than we are deciding that it's okay to do to us what we, as humankind, do to animals. Would we not object? When an entity that is presumed by many to be larger than we are as individuals (i.e., presidential administrations, organizations like the FDA, etc.) makes decisions that impact our fates in ways that we don't approve of or agree with, we have the intelligence and opportunity to protest. And we *do*. Every single day.

We have dominion over animals. That does not mean we have the right to harm what is under our dominion at will or neglect taking action against the entities that bring them harm. From both a religious and secular position, it is the exact opposite of that. As we are given dominion over the animals of our lands, we become caretakers of creation. If we care about our own *children*, whom we, as adults, naturally have dominion over, does that not also apply to the animal kingdom?

But we already have so many animal rights groups out there tending to this. There are laws protecting animals all over the place. Doesn't it seem clear that we are doing what we can already?

For many, yes. But some still lack one important distinction in their approach to concern for animals.

While it is true that our civilization largely frowns upon the direct and malicious abuse of animals as it even appears in our legislation regarding animal rights, it's not enough that it's merely illegal on paper to intentionally hurt an animal. This serves to create a sense of responsibility that responds only to an outright attack. Such acute focus is not conducive to ideal health or welfare. That is comparable to a parent intervening on his or her child's behalf only when imminent threat or abuse presents itself, instead of seeing to that child's need for love, attention, and health in all other areas of growth and development. So, to those who believe we're doing our part by refusing to tolerate direct abuse, these authors beg the readers to reassess their role in not only caring for animals, but in loving and prioritizing them also.

Is this to suggest that I should give my pet the same priority as other humans or my own family?

No.

One important distinction begs to be addressed for the sake of balance. Many of us would give every dime we have to save one of our children or beloved family members. We would gladly take a bullet, jump in front of a moving bus, or lay down our lives in any way in order to keep them alive and well. But if a family pet were to become sick, we may not be willing to die, go bankrupt, or deplete our family's savings accounts to send the pet to an advanced-level university hospital to try to save them if they develop some rare or complicated illness, even though we care about them and don't wish them any pain. Does that make us immoral? No, it doesn't, and here's why: Whereas we should always treat animals with respect, we should never place the welfare of our animals above other human beings. Would one spend five hundred dollars saving a single animal? Many of us would, or at least we would try if we had the means. Would one spend five hundred *thousand* dollars saving a single animal? Many would not. If we had five hundred thousand extra dollars lying around, it may do the human race a lot more good being donated to the Doernbecher's Hospital for Pediatric Cancer Research. And that decision, like all others to protect an animal or feed the continual well-being of humanity, would be up to the individual.

There certainly *is* a greater responsibility toward the care of humans. This is a given, and any reader of this book should know that these authors are not suggesting otherwise. But with that said, there will always be a responsibility in placing our potential as human caretakers over the animal kingdom when it fits into our capacity to do so. If the line were ever drawn between placing our potential to save a child versus our potential to save an animal, then we can and *should* choose the child. Yet, if the resources are there to do both, we have a duty to do both. We should not tolerate a society that shrugs with indifference upon the mistreatment of animals when our capabilities of showing compassion to them are accessible. But our society *can and does* tolerate the abuse of animals, and the proof is everywhere, least of all in a small study of FDA regulations (such as that which follows this chapter). In doing so, we draw a line that should never be drawn. To the extent that it is within our power to care for and protect all of creation— humans, animals, plants—it would be immoral not to. The fact that our world will approve a certain treatment of animals with an approach that has been forbidden within the scope of high standard human living says something about the disconnect in our mindset between humans as a dominating species over the lesser.

This does not mean that you should join a radical animal rights group. This does not mean that the world would be a better place if all humans were exterminated so that the animals could have their own Shangri-La. As awareness is raised regarding the mistreatment of animals, the world has begun moving toward a higher level of respect toward them, one step at a time. This book is merely a tool to bring further appreciation and knowledge to the categories of mistreatment that still rage on daily, with a central focus on food.

Now, let's begin our reflection of the regulation deficiencies we encounter within the pet food industry.

Chapter Two

The "Pass-the-Buck" Regulation Game

There is no requirement that pet food products
have pre-market approval by the FDA.
—Official FDA Website[11]

Many people assume that the products they purchase off the shelf at a grocery store have been rigorously tested by some government agency or association for safety before they ever become available to consumers. Regarding pet food specifically, some may assume the United States Department of Agriculture (USDA) monitors pet food ingredients via their Food Safety and Inspection Service or Animal and Plant Health Inspection Service. In fact, the USDA's services monitor the humane treatment of animals and inspect some foods intended for human consumption, but they have absolutely nothing to do with pet food ingredients.

Who Regulates?

With the USDA ruled out, we are left with the Food and Drug Administration (FDA), the Association of American Feed Control Officials (AAFCO), and the Pet Food Institute (PFI).

FDA

The writers of this book acknowledge that there are well-meaning individuals within the FDA who honestly strive toward the goal of monitoring the safety of the food consumed by both pets and humans. However, as a whole, the FDA falls shockingly short of delivering safety to both American citizens and their beloved pets.

Books have been written for years discussing the inadequacies of the FDA concerning nutrition regulation. The research is plentiful and accessible by anyone, yet when the facts are exposed, people seem shocked. Why do people believe that we are being taken care of? To answer that, we will quickly refer to the quote by Adolf Hitler mentioned in the previous chapter: "If you tell a big enough lie and tell it frequently enough, it will be believed."

So, the FDA is lying to us?

Not always, and not directly. They are, however, wise enough to understand that the average pet owner is not going to have the law degree required to comprehend the complexities of all the hundreds of pages of legalese they give public access to. An extremely bright person may have a very hard time researching why Fido is suddenly ill based on the lack of FDA regulations. Almost anything can be said out in the open, and it can even be said honestly: If an entity shrouds the truth in enough thorny language, most people can't follow it.

To begin, there is not enough staff or time available for the FDA to give the proper attention to every ingredient that goes into human or pet consumables. Marion Nestle, investigative author of *Pet Food Politics: The Chihuahua in the Coal Mine*, reported the following:

> To speak only of food inspections: the United States currently imports about 80% of its seafood, 32% of its fruit and nuts, 13% of its vegetables, and 10% of its meats. In 2007, these foods arrived in 25,000 shipments a day from about 100 countries. The FDA was able to inspect only about 1% of these shipments, down from 8% in 1992. In contrast, the USDA is able to inspect 16% of the foods under its purview. By one assessment, the FDA has become so short-staffed that it would take the agency 1,900 years to inspect every foreign [manufacturing/rendering] plant that exports food to the United States.[12]

Almost immediately, it becomes all too obvious that the FDA can't monitor all of our people foods and pet foods— even if they wanted to. Of the imported foods listed above, the FDA only inspected 1 percent of twenty-five thousand shipments of imported foods in a single day! If Fido were promised to live almost two thousand years, we wouldn't have a problem, because that's all the time that the FDA would need to inspect all the foreign sources they allow into our country. Given that our pets' clocks on this earth were already ticking well before you even purchased this book, we have some digging to do, and fast.

But the issues with the FDA monitoring aren't limited to the lack of time and people needed to do the job. Some things they take time to test and be entirely aware of they choose to completely ignore. Take, for instance, this example: From the FDA website, salmonella (a dangerous bacterium from the same family as E. coli that causes illnesses such as typhoid fever and food poisoning) and listeria monocytogenes (a bacterium that causes the infection listeriosis, an attack against the central nervous system) were found in 196 samples from fifteen commercial dog and cat foods from October 2010 through July 2012.[13] Yet, despite the extreme threat these bacteria posed to cats and dogs, the FDA did not issue a recall.[14] Those who have suggested that the FDA does not have the authority to take action, the FDA clearly states on their website: "FDA does not approve pet food, but rather approves the food additives that are used in pet food. *FDA has the authority to take action against pet food products that are in violation of the law.*"[15] It doesn't take a scientist in a lab coat to hypothesize that knowingly allowing the distribution of food sources causing food-borne illnesses is against the law.

Surely, this example is an oversight. Right? But if it were, would it happen continuously? Not to mention, they write and disobey their own policies on the protein by-products that go into the foods. (More on the FDA's inconsistencies about protein by-products in the next chapter.)

Straight from the FDA's own website:

> There is *no requirement that pet food products have pre-market approval by the FDA*. However, FDA ensures that the ingredients used in pet food are safe and have an appropriate function in the pet food. *Many ingredients such as meat, poultry and grains are considered safe and do not require pre-market approval.* Other substances such as sources of minerals, vitamins or other nutrients, flavorings, preservatives, or processing aids may be generally recognized as safe (GRAS) for an intended use (21 CFR 582 and 584) or must have approval as food additives (21 CFR 570, 571 and 573). Colorings must have approvals for that use as specified in 21 CFR 70 and be listed in Parts 73, 74, or 81.[16]

Many ingredients like meat are considered safe? They don't require pre-market approval? And what is "pre-market" approval? Apparently, it's "a review of safety and effectiveness by FDA experts and agency approval before a product can be marketed." And yet, the FDA says that isn't necessary for pet foods or ingredients such as meat, poultry, and grains that go into pet foods.

Remember when you were little and your parents always instructed you to be careful about meat? These authors do.

We were told things like, "Make sure to always heat that in the microwave until it's piping hot! It has meat in it. It can be dangerous if it's not fully cooked [or heated]." Or, if a meat was a few days old or older: "I wouldn't eat that if I were you. That meat has been there a while." Or when handling raw meat: "Make sure to really wash and get all that raw meat off your hands. Those germs can kill ya." Meat, when handled properly and when sourced from a safe animal, holds fantastic nutrient components in a well-balanced diet for both humans and pets. When sourced from an animal in unsafe conditions or mishandled (such as the protein sources we will be addressing in this book), it can be very dangerous. Pets can become ill as a result of bad food just like people can.

So does the FDA ensure safety, or not? Actually, you may be surprised to hear that they have less to do with regulation than you thought, if you read farther into the complicated and confusing policies listed on the "FDA's Regulation of Pet Food" page:

> A food additive petition is the pre-clearance mechanism developed by the FDA for demonstrating that a food additive is safe for its intended use and has utility. If the FDA agrees with the petition, a regulation is published in the *Federal Register* and 21 CFR, Part 573, Food Additives Permitted in the Feed and Drinking Water of Animals, is amended.... Briefly, a petition contains a description of the chemical identity, manufacturing process and controls, analytical methods, utility data, human food safety data, target

animal safety data, product labeling, and in some cases an environmental assessment.[17]

Here we read that the FDA requires a "food additive petition," wherein a "description" of the chemical and manufacturing processes is given, as well as a "description" of how the data of the additive meets the standards for pet safety, and sometimes (or "in some cases") they assess the environment. There's a lot of slack here. The organization goes on to say:

> CVM [Center for Veterinary Medicine, a branch of the FDA] has used regulatory discretion and *not required food additive petitions for substances that do not raise any safety concerns.* In this case, *we ask the company to submit the information needed* to list the ingredient in the Official Publication of the Association of American Feed Control Officials (AAFCO).[18]

By their own admission, it appears that the "food additive petition" that involves "descriptions" of safety isn't even required by the FDA in the first place, unless safety issues arise. To these authors, that sounds like regulation isn't required until regulation becomes required. Wonderfully circular logic. And, if safety issues have not yet been raised, *the company* is allowed to submit the ingredient to AAFCO for inclusion in its official publication. The *company?* Surely a company with greedy pockets screaming for monetary gain wouldn't stretch the truth just to make a buck…

But we digress. Let's continue down the FDA trail:

This ingredient definition process [the "food additive petition"] is done to conserve agency resources, as food additive approval is *time-consuming*. [Remember the quote above about 1,900 years. Now here, they admit to cutting corners.] CVM reviews the data [you know, that "described" data] to ensure the ingredient has utility and can be manufactured consistently to meet product specifications. Although ingredients used under regulatory discretion are still *unapproved food additives*, we agree *we will not take regulatory action as long as the labeling is consistent with the accepted intended use, the labeling or advertising does not make drug claims, and new data are not received that raise questions concerning safety or suitability.*[19]

The FDA "will not take regulatory action" for pet foods, even with "unapproved food additives" as long as the label looks good, nobody claims the food has healing properties or special drugs intended to improve an animal's condition, and no new information pops up showing the food is unsafe? (Unless, of course, like in the example above, salmonella and listeria monocytogenes bacteria are found in the foods. In that case, the FDA probably won't do anything about it.)

To gain further insight and understanding of this whole process and the holes therein, we contacted the CEO of a holistic soap company, Allie Anderson of Eden's Essentials, in hopes that she would help provide a comparison for our readers, using soap-cooking as an example.[20] If the authors of this book understand all of this correctly—as well as other authors who have studied the inner workings of the FDA and written books, blogs, articles, and dissertations about how they are greatly lacking in regulation—this following example appears to be an accurate comparison to the moral code regarding pet foods (note that these authors are not claiming this exact scenario has happened or would happen in association with any existing soap company or products):

- Sarah decides to start a "healthy, holistic soap company" using various scents, colors, ingredients, and appeal that target specific buyers. The soap she chooses to target to mothers with infants has a helpful ingredient, Melaleuca Alternifolia—tea tree oil—a common oil used to treat diaper rash. (According to WebMD, it is also commonly used to treat acne, fungal infections, athlete's foot, and ringworm. As an antiseptic, it can be used for burns, cuts, bug bites, vaginal infections, and herpes.[21])
- Although Sarah shares that her baby soap contains an ingredient known to assist the skin in faster healing, she makes sure that the soap is not being marketed as a drug, nor does she make any claims that the soap has any specific healing properties. This ensures that she is properly abiding by the FDA's regulation of labeling accuracy, and advertising that the appropriate "intent of use" and "utility" in relation to the intended function of the soap is merely to "Lather, rinse, and give your baby the best!" (Sound familiar?)

- "According to research conducted by the National Institutes of Health's National Institute of Environmental Health Sciences (NIEHS)," tea tree oil used on infants *may* cause prepubertal gynecomastia, a condition "resulting in enlarged breast tissue in prepubescent boys."[22] (Additionally, the oil can cause rashes and boils on someone who is allergic.) Sarah knows this, but chooses to make the soap anyway, because *her* company's soap will differ from her competitors and look better on the product label (becoming our proverbial "greedy company" for this comparative example).

- Sarah launches an ad campaign involving television commercials showing happy babies thriving and crawling across the floor with healthy skin, giggling, and interacting with their caring parents, suggesting that their choice of soap has improved their baby's life.

- As Sarah continues to make money on her soap scheme, little boys are developing extra breast tissue, and allergic infants whose mothers wanted to help clear up their diaper rash are developing more rashes and boils than before. Confused parents don't conclude immediately that their young boy with chest protrusions or their little girl with an increasing rash problem had anything to do with the "holistic" soap they were using. Why not? Because tea tree oil is an ingredient largely associated with healing properties, and they don't think to research that specific ingredient. Even if they *do* conclude that the soap they are using on their child may be causing an allergic reaction, they chalk it up to their baby being allergic to that specific soap, and not to tea tree oil. It takes years, *if at all*, for parents to make this association, and by then, the damage to the boy's chest or the chaos of rashes on the skin has already been endured, and it's likely that the FDA was never even notified.

• Because safety issues never officially or publicly arose, Sarah continues to make and distribute her harmful product.

In case you are wondering, tea tree oil is *not* "generally recognized as safe" (or "GRAS") according to the FDA; they stated this in a recent warning letter to a company called Ad-Med Bio-technology, LLC, concerning a drug product.[23] The FDA seems to have very little to say about it, actually. From the WebMD site on tea tree oil, we read: "[The FDA] does not regulate tea tree oil in the same way it regulates medicines. *It can be sold with limited or no research on how well it works.*"[24] Despite this, you may be surprised to hear that *hundreds* of tea tree oil soaps, body washes, and shampoos are available on the market that claim to be FDA-approved, *or* that contain only FDA-approved ingredients, several of which are marketed directly for use on infants' skin and hair. (Google this to see all the brands for yourself. We have not researched each of these soaps to see if anything on the warning label gives parents a heads-up not to use it on their children, because, as we said above, this was merely an example. That said, there is much research to support the idea that this oil is incredibly healthy for many uses.)

But who decides if something is safe or "GRAS"?

"[The] FDA is charged with the enforcement of the Federal Food, Drug, and Cosmetic Act (the Act),"[25] as they admit on their website. Farther down, we read this:

> As interpreted by FDA and the courts, there are two requirements that must be satisfied before a substance can be GRAS—general recognition and safety:
> 1. For general recognition, there must be an expert consensus that the substance is safe for use as a component of food, and;
> 2. This expert consensus of safety must be based on either (a) generally available data and information to show common use of the substance in animal feed prior to 1958 or (b) scientific procedures, which require the same quantity and quality of scientific data needed for FDA approval of the substance as a food additive. In addition, this information must be published in the scientific literature.[26]

So, setting aside for a moment that anything "prior to 1958" would be exceedingly outdated to our modern world with ever-changing and evolving pet breeds, we see that the food must be considered safe by "expert" consensus (this looks promising) *or* "scientific procedures." If a man in a lab coat says it's safe, then it is. Oh, *and* the information must be published in scientific literature. But, didn't we already discover that being published in scientific literature was as easy as the greedy company submitting paperwork to AAFCO? In fact, it seems like that's all there is to it. Observe what the FDA says about the GRAS determination:

> The Act ["the Federal Food, Drug, and Cosmetic Act"] *permits companies to make their own GRAS determination* [so the man in the lab coat can work for the company?], and many times GRAS Panels will be assembled that are comprised of scientific experts in a particular field to evaluate the safety of a substance for an intended use. However, *regardless of who makes the determination, the FDA or the company*, the standard for GRAS is the same.[27]

If a greedy company is able to make its own "generally considered as safe" determination in so many cases, why do we need the FDA? Additionally, it looks like "any person" can inform the FDA that the use of a substance is GRAS, and the FDA *will not* conduct their own evaluation:

> On April 17, 1997, the Center for Food Safety and Applied Nutrition (CFSAN) and CVM published a proposed rule in the Federal Register (62 FR 18938) to amend the regulations to *replace the current GRAS affirmation process with a notification procedure.* Under the notification procedure, *any person could notify the agency of a determination that a particular use of a substance is GRAS.* The notification would include a description of the substance, the conditions of use, and

the basis of the GRAS determination. *The FDA would not conduct its own detailed evaluation of the data*, as was done previously for GRAS affirmation petitions.[28]

Taking all of this into consideration, registering a complaint to the FDA over a sick pet should, according to their own words above, result in action against a pet food company that has made a pet sick by selling unsafe or un-GRAS food. Right? Actually, it's far more complicated than that.

Ann Martin, international pet food authority and author of *Food Pets Die For: Shocking Facts about Pet Food* and *Protect Your Pet: More Shocking Facts*, has been a well known whistle-blower of the dangers behind commercial pet foods for well over a decade. Her unprecedented research into the blatant failings of safety regulations in the FDA (and their associates) is unmatched. Her persistent questions to the authorities on regulations have been documented. According to Martin, if a pet owner should contact the FDA concerning a sick or dying pet with claims that the food commercially available was responsible for the pet's condition, the owner meets great resistance. As she states in *Food Pets Die For*, the FDA must be provided with "chemical analysis" of the food the pet has been fed (very convoluted intel for a consumer to gather, to be sure), as well as veterinary documentation including "any blood work, urinalysis, and any other medical tests done on your pet."[29] And, as Martin goes on to say, these test requirements are astronomically expensive to produce. We can safely assume that many people will let the issue drop here, requiring no further investigation by the FDA. (Using our earlier soap company comparison, if concerned parents want to take action against "Sarah" because of what her tea tree soap has done to an infant, they may have to be very wealthy in order to accomplish this by these standards.)

AAFCO

It appears that the FDA relies a great deal on AAFCO for ideal pet food practice. However, there are several key factors readers must know about AAFCO. Again, the authors of this book are aware that there are many great people within this association who work diligently to see pet food standards held high, but their role is sadly negligible as far as accomplishing regulation. One of the first things seen at the top of the home page of the organization's official website, just under the heading, "Purpose and Function of AAFCO," is that "AAFCO has no regulatory authority."[30]

Their role as a helpful nongovernment organization is to "provide a forum" for "local, state, and federal agencies" to come together and write up model laws "regulating the manufacture, distribution and sale of animal feeds."[31] But without the authority to regulate or enforce on their end, all they can do is provide "good idea" laws and "suggest" that the entities that *do* have the authority to regulate follow them. At the end of the day—and we mean this with no disrespect for the good deeds the organization does accomplish—for the purposes of pet food regulation, they appear to simply be a lot of nice people suggesting a lot of nice things with no authority to execute wholesome convictions.

Throughout the years, as AAFCO's business models and policies have evolved, there have been whispers that AAFCO will conduct their own pet food testing, reserving their official seal of approval for only those brands that meet their requirements. However, shoppers hoping to find the "AAFCO Approved" sticker on the front of dog food bags will be disappointed. Their website makes this very clear:

> **AAFCO does not regulate, test, approve or certify pet foods in any way.**
>
> AAFCO establishes the nutritional standards for complete and balanced pet foods, and *it is the pet food company's responsibility* to formulate their products according to the appropriate AAFCO standard.[32]

So, if every pet food company in the United States were run by caring, honest people who never cut corners and were always willing to hire the most proficient scientific personnel in order to spare no expense in assuring that every last batch of food was up to AAFCO standards, we wouldn't have a problem. But, this far into the study, we already know that we can't rely on the FDA *or* AAFCO to check up on these companies. Common sense, along with all the animals dying as a result of death-causing ingredients, tells us that major money-making companies absolutely can and will cut corners wherever and however they can to make an extra buck and spare additional research and labor, as well as alleviate the need to keep up on the most recent changes in laws and regulations.

Since it appears that no action against the companies will be taken unless the food raises safety concerns, they can continue to let their standards drop well below AAFCO's suggested practice. Since it appears that no safety concerns will be raised unless a pet owner has the financial wherewithal to launch a huge investigation on his own time and confront the FDA directly with irrefutable and documented proof that his pet's death and/or illness with vet bills was a result of said company, the FDA will not get involved. Since AAFCO has no authority and the FDA won't exercise their authority, why would we draw any other conclusion than that rich companies are exploiting consumers?

Could the Pet Food Institute do something, maybe?

PFI

At the onset, the Pet Food Institute appears to be very intertwined with regulatory endeavors and associated closely with both the FDA and AAFCO in the interest of keeping pet foods standards as high as possible. However, much like AAFCO, their hands are tied where authority or action is concerned. On the organization's official website, on the "Most Highly Regulated" page under the "Pet Food Info" category, one of the first things they admit is having no regulatory authority: "Pet food labeling and advertising claims are regulated by the federal government and by the states."[33] From that comment forward, the web page speaks nothing more of PFI's involvement and redirects the reader's attention to what AAFCO strives to do. On the "About PFI" page, we read what they are truly responsible for:

Since 1958, PFI has been the voice of the makers of U.S. cat and dog food. Driven by an active and dedicated membership, PFI is the industry's public and media relations resource, representative before state and federal agencies, organizer of seminars and educational programs, sponsor of and clearinghouse for research, and liaison with other organizations.

For more than 55 years, PFI has worked with its members to educate the owners of cats and dogs about pet nutrition and health.[34]

To view PFI with anything less than respect would be a great injustice to *some* of its members, as their role primarily has been to educate people about how to better care for their animals' needs—and this is an honorable enterprise. However, note that there is much conspiracy in PFI's membership bias. There are two categories of membership within PFI: "active" and "affiliate." The "active" members are primarily made up of commercial pet food manufacturers, and the "affiliate" members include leadership and owners behind some of the largest rendering plants in the country. (More about rendering plants in the next chapter.) This would mean, of course, that PFI is largely established from a biased group of individuals who strive to educate people about pet food safety, but it appears that the education people are receiving points back to *their* pet foods being the best. Is this a coincidence? In addition, they are located in Washington DC, where they have close access to influencing legislation.

The Evolution of Law

Nonetheless, sadly, because PFI is more of a knowledge base for the public to begin their own research and not a magical entity with the power to wave a magic wand and reconstruct/repair the fallacies of the industry, we land at the same conclusion: AAFCO can't do anything; PFI can't do anything; FDA won't do anything because they are relying on everyone else to follow the unregulated and nonmandatory guidelines "suggested" by associations like AAFCO and PFI, unless safety concerns have been raised as a result of massive public outcry or a victim wealthy enough to provide scientific and medical documentation before, during, and after his bouts with the harmful food/product. Because many consumers do not link their pets' illnesses or health symptoms to diet or pharmaceuticals because their bag of chow features a picture of a happy guy in a lab coat with perfect teeth and dapper hair giving the thumbs-up gesture to the buyer—indicating that this brand of dog food is perfectly balanced and healthy, and therefore couldn't possibly cause any health issues (you know, that "scientist" whom "the company" hired)—public outcry is not likely to occur. Instead, many pet owners receive the sad news from their vet that Fido has to be put down because of cancer or organ failure, and well, "these things happen"…

Essentially, we could spend another five hundred pages talking about the varying associations, companies, governmental administrations, and well-meaning organizations, and continue to come back around to this sad conclusion.

On the surface, and primarily for the last sixty years, laws regarding animal feed and pet foods have continued to be amended and in some cases changed altogether. From time to time, encouraging movements occur on a national level to spread awareness and lift the standards of industry practice. As an example: Most recently, the launch of the AFRPS (Animal Feed Regulatory Program Standards), a collaboration between the FDA and AAFCO, boosted confidence in the system. This new program for state animal feed regulators includes enticing and hopeful verbiage relating to overall higher and more efficient "standards that serve as an objective framework to evaluate and improve components of a State feed program. The standards cover the State feed program's regulatory foundation, training, inspection program, auditing, feed-related illness or death and emergency response, enforcement program, outreach activities, budget and planning, laboratory services, sampling program, and assessment and improvement of standard implementation."[35] To a casual observer, a high five is in order, as it appears that the FDA has finally launched something that will raise the bar—on a state level at least. However, regrettably, this program, also, is not mandatory in any way. Just above these encouraging words we've just read is a simple and demoralizing statement: "Implementation of the AFRPS is *voluntary.*"[36] (Not to mention this little zinger, just below within the same document, which raises the question of when official "suggestions" will ever stop being a part of our federal regulations: "The term 'should' is used throughout the AFRPS. Program elements and corresponding conditions described as 'should' are best practices but *are optional and not required to fully implement a standard.*"[37])

When we read about programs like these, we find ourselves excited about the implications that our country's animals will live longer, more comfortable lives as a result of proper training and increased awareness of healthier practices from the federal level down. It appears that perhaps the nation is finally moving in the right direction. But is it ever, really? Or is this the latest round of smoke and mirrors? The latest round of feel-good movements giving the "green" activists reason to believe that something is being done? The latest round of flashy, wordy, complicated documents offering to placate audiences who are demanding an explanation from the FDA?

Whether programs like these are genuine efforts or another series of papers attempting to pressure the government to act on it is not something that these authors can conclude for certain. In either case, the fact that these programs are surfacing now more frequently than they did historically shows an increase in the number of, and action taken by, those who care.

Yet, after seeing words like "voluntary" and "should" being associated with so many of our federal paper trails, it's simple to see that we still haven't arrived at a higher level of regulation for Fido's protection. Laws and legislation corresponding to foods and medicines in the US evolve rapidly, frequently, and dramatically. What was true yesterday will be updated tomorrow; what is true tomorrow will be negated by new laws and information available in fifty years. For all we know, by the time this book has reached you, the laws and programs will already be altered. And though there will always be well-meaning and sincere individuals within activist or regulatory associations, there will also always be those looking to cut corners and fool the public into thinking we are all taken care of, whether the reason for their deception stems from pure laziness or something more complicated and beyond their control, like the lack of funding, time, resources, and/or staff to keep the standards high. The responsibility of animal feeding really always has (and maybe always will) belonged to you: the animal's owner.

Now, with the main three organizations most associated with regulation addressed, let's focus upon the veterinarian's role in all of this.

Ask Your Veterinarian?

By now, many readers are likely thinking that they can rely on their veterinarians to direct them to the most healthy and breed-appropriate food and medicine sources. These are not only the brands/products that the professionals recommend, they are the brands/products carried at the office with the vets' hearty stamp of approval as they offer warm handshakes. It's more personal, more *trustworthy*, than the picture of the unknown man in the lab coat on the front of the bag at the store. Who wouldn't feel reassured purchasing everything Fido needs directly from that really nice vet who patted your pup on the head when you walked into his office instead of off the shelves in a standard grocery aisle? Whereas your vet is a very good place to start your research, it's certainly not always a good idea to rely solely on veterinary recommendations above and beyond your own ability to examine the facts.

There are many honest, well-meaning veterinary professionals who have a sincere interest in the well-being of animals. If they weren't interested in keeping Fido healthy, they wouldn't have dedicated their lives to that ideal in the first place, right? This is true in many cases. In the end, the authenticity behind a personal recommendation from an animal healthcare professional must rely on two things: 1) the trust/relationship between the veterinarian and the pet owner; and 2) the pet owner's personal knowledge of harmful pet food/medicine ingredients. It never hurts to consider the advice of professionals who appear to care about a pet's health, but it also never hurts to verify the information they give via your own research.

Some veterinarians—*most often those belonging to larger clinics with numerous staff, which gain more attention from product manufacturers*—have their own reasoning for giving their nod of approval or wave of dismissal toward specific pet food brands and/or medical products (flea collars, heartworm treatments, dandruff shampoos, etc.) unrelated to the quality of the product. These products, both prescription and non-prescription, often aren't any healthier or more impressive nutritionally or medically (or more regulated on the manufacturing level) than the cheapest goods on the shelf at a regular grocery store, though their prices are frequently inflated several times over. Pet owners, such as pet food authority Ann

Martin, find the idea of vet clinics selling pet foods offensive, because holding a degree or certificate in veterinary practice (the caring for ill or injured animals) is nothing close to the same as being an expert in nutrition. Certainly, a veterinarian would know more about the certain food-related effects on an animal's anatomy than a layman, but, to summarize an argument Martin eloquently unfolded in *Food Pets Die For*: For the same reason we do not find diabetes-fighting food, life-stage appropriate food, and kidney-disease-fighting foods (etc.) on the shelves of our family doctor's office, because they are there to treat illness or injury—*despite* the fact that they are more knowledgeable about the effects food has on human anatomy than their patients are—we should not find pet foods at a vet clinic.[38]

Occasionally called "kickbacks," food and medicine companies sometimes offer monetary rewards for vet professionals who endorse their brands. The vets' incentive to push these products can be driven far more by greed than by their belief in value of these goods. In addition to the personal gain, there can be a "team reward" assigned to the entire veterinary clinic at the end of the year if an office achieves a certain sales number. So, to the individual with moral conviction—who would not regularly participate in pitching junk products to his clientele for extra pocket jingle—there is understandably much pressure to participate in the scheme "as a team" for the benefit of the clinic. If the sales bonus requirement is not met for that office, the annual incentive check is not rewarded, all because those who didn't believe the program was ethical or honest (or they were poor salespeople, too lazy, etc.) ruined it for the rest of them. As the need/want for additional annual income increases for the staff, the pressure builds upon the clientele/pet owners to purchase the product, which naturally prompts the passionate delivery of the endorsement at the time of the sale, sometimes leading to the stretching of the truth, as some morally wanting salespeople will say whatever they need to in the moment in order to put another checkmark on their sales sheet. When questioned about where they obtain their knowledge about the food they are pitching, they typically say they got it from classes, seminars, lectures, etc.—which sounds reassuring, until the consumer later discovers that *most* of these classes are taught by representatives of the companies that manufacture the food (naturally biased and not altogether honest sources).[39]

Some claim that these incentive programs are utter nonsense, and chalk them all up to sensational conspiracy. Others admit openly that at one point in their career or as a student of the veterinary field, they have participated in biased sales pitching for bonus checks. The reason for such varying declarations is most likely a result of the companies' targeted clinics. If a nice man in the middle of nowhere runs his own practice with a single assistant from the nearby town at the front desk, he doesn't draw as much attention for potential sales ranks. If a huge, fully-staffed veterinary office with multiple practitioners is attending to large numbers of patients in a big city, the manufacturers of food/medical products are likely paying closer attention and giving reason for these clinics to endorse their goods. This is mutually beneficial, as the vet professionals receive rewards and the manufacturers earn a higher status as the makers of the brands "recommended by vets." (This is not to assume that any small clinic is immune to dishonesty or that any larger clinic automatically participates in deceitfulness or scams.)

Keep in mind that not only is there nothing wrong with product mark-ups in a clinic, it simply makes good business sense to make money where money can be made. Because animal health clinics are not pet stores, naturally, the products they carry will be more expensive than the goods would be in a local feed or grocery store (due to lower volumes of sales at the clinic, shipping, cost of operation in a medical setting versus retail, etc.). Thus, one should not assume that a clinic is participating in a dirty scheme just because it stocks a certain item at a higher price than a retail store.

If you are unsure of your vet clinic's motivation for carrying certain brands, it is within your right to ask whether the clinic is participating in an incentive program. However, because there are many professionals who do operate transparently and honestly for the good of your animal, offer these inquiries with respect. As a result of the public's increased awareness of these programs in recent decades, sometimes a vet's recommendation is instantly written off because a pet owner is skeptical of the motive, resulting in said pet owner traveling to a local pet store for an "unbiased" opinion. Ultimately, the logic behind this action is faulty, since retail stores are operated by people with far less knowledge of an animal's needs than a veterinary professional. It makes no sense to leave a vet clinic for fear of corrupt sales motives to get a product recommendation from a layman who works nine to five at a pet store. The best route to obtaining the healthiest goods for Fido involves a combination of self-education and a relationship with a professional who can be trusted.

Chapter Three

Where's the Beef?!

We are healthy only to the extent
that our ideas are humane.
—KURT VONNEGUT[40]

It's easy to assume that we have been in the pet food business for hundreds of years, and that by now we would have figured out how to go about it safely. However, the business of pet foods has only been a part of our world for a very short time. Currently, billions of dollars per year are spent in the US alone to give our animal companions feed, specialized diets, treats, etc., but it wasn't until the 1960s that the production of pet foods became a *widespread* commercial endeavor. In the 1800s, the first commercially marketed "dog cakes" (dog biscuits), invented by James Spratt, consisted of meat, vegetables, and wheat meals, and were sold in the US circa 1890. Prior to this, table scraps were the only pet food, and despite new and innovative feeding ideas, it would take nearly a century for common households to latch on to the idea of feeding pets with anything but our own leftovers.

Apart from Spratt's efforts, it was not until WWII that commercial pet food became a national enterprise. At this point, the primary source of protein was the meat from deceased horses. By the end of the war, our nation was spending $200 million per year on pet foods, and in the glamorous 1930s, canned cat foods became a lucrative market. As technology slowly replaced horses in the farming industry, horse meat became less and less a central ingredient for pet foods, replaced instead with grains and protein by-products, with little to no concern from the trusting public as to the origin of the ingredients. (After all, it wasn't like we were talking about what *humans* would be consuming; it was just cats and dogs, a different species from we fragile homo sapiens, and they were impervious to the illnesses a human could get from improperly handled or suspect food sources... Or, at least that was the thought process at the time the earliest pet food chains were established.)

In the 1950s, Spratt's merged with General Mills, and within the following decade, a great cat and dog food variety hit the shelves, available for anyone with Fidos and Fluffys cuddled up at their hearths. Radio and television commercials began developing catchy jingles, and for the first time in human-animal companionship history, our pets had earned representation in the major media as "a part of the family." When bell bottoms, burnt-orange blazers, and olive green polyester vests erupted in fashion departments during the flower-child generation of the earth-loving 70s, alongside them came an array of colorful pet food labels appealing to more discriminating needs. These included specialized diets for kittens and puppies, formulas for weight-challenged pets, feeds for specific breeds, and the start of a stiff competition between companies to see which brands claimed to contain the most meat.

Discussions of "healthy" pet foods were now popping up nationally, but for the most part, only the wealthiest and the most concerned Americans would spring for the pricier foods purported to meet their animals' individual needs, because the concept of caring about a feline or canine as a "member of the family" was still in its infancy. Many dogs and cats were still being fed whatever hadn't been consumed by their masters during family dinners, and those who chose to provide their pets with their own bag or can of food typically didn't see the need to buy anything more impressive than the most generic and affordable options.

By the 1980s, celebrity endorsements became the norm; advertisements represented a deeper connection between humans and animals: They were buddies and comrades instead of masters and property. Pets as "members of the family" or "man's best friend" were at long last respected by the general public; and most households finally adopted the idea of buying Fido his own chow.

Some passionate, modern-day pet health and wellness advocates question why we have not yet perfected the production and regulation of pet foods, reasoning that we have been at this pet-food making business long enough to know better than to fall prey to clever company schemes or buy food without knowing how to read a label. And whereas their zeal toward these and other similar goals are commendable, our nation simply hasn't prioritized animals for as long as it may seem to our current generation. Because of voices like theirs and books like this, our country has started to take a second glance at what goes into the feeding tray. To the pet owners of the 70s and 80s, it was a great service to our companions just to toss the foods designed for their species into the shopping cart in the first place.

In regards to the mindset of the general population of America (as well as other countries prosperous enough to consider pet companion health), society wasn't willing and ready to arm ourselves to the teeth with cries of war against the injustice of unhealthy ingredients in pet foods until very recently. Aside from society's mentality regarding the respect of animals as companions, with each major breakthrough in veterinary medicine and canine/feline diet-related research and development, we reach new milestones in broadening the awareness of what their bodies *can* and *can't* safely receive. Because table scraps came off of our own plates, they were originally fit for the high standards of human consumption, and our proteins were mostly farm-raised and grass-fed. Without the preservatives and harmful chemicals added to current pet foods, the general public's knowledge of what pets should be eating was experimental at best when comparing the new industry practice to today's practice. To the pet food production lines fired up in the 1930s, meat was just meat, grains were just grains, and that was all there was to it.

It has taken our society decades of pet illness and veterinary intervention to arrive at weeding out the bad foods from the safe foods, and we are merely at the cusp, only just now, of raising an all-new awareness of what should and shouldn't be in products that have pictures of happy dogs and fluffy kittens on the packaging. The infancy of our previous concern (that of the individual as well as of major regulation deficiencies)—added to the certain companies and personalities that can and will cut corners in the privacy of their manufacturing plants, all while giving a warm and reassuring smile to the public—is a perfect recipe for allowing unhealthy pet foods to become the norm.

We *are* getting there. But until we do arrive at a healthier food-processing reality for our pets, some very shocking things are going on in the business of pet foods. So far, we have discussed the overall lack of regulation that leads to terrible food-handling and cooking processes, but we haven't yet discussed what, exactly, lurks in those foods that are killing our household companions.

WARNING: Although the authors of this book have gone out of their way to omit graphic material, by nature, a lot of what will be discussed in the following pages is disgusting, and the details we must mention in order to inform a reading audience could be disturbing to some. Readers' discretion is advised.

Rendering Plants: It's a Dog-Eat-Dead-Dog World

Directly from *Dogs Naturally Magazine*:

> This is old news for many but it bears repeating. If you feed commercial pet foods, you had better do your research and find out exactly what is in that food....

"Would it surprise you to learn that what your beloved pets have been eating is at least partly made of euthanized pets?"

It's true. The companies that do their best to convince us that they have our pets' best interests at heart and produce dog and cat food packages showing juicy cuts of real beef, lamb, chicken and fish, are actually packing those cans and bags full of dead animals of every sort: diseased cattle, tumor-ridden chickens, road kill, zoo animals, and even, yes, dogs and cats from veterinarians and shelters around the country, not to mention rancid restaurant grease, toxic chemicals and other unsavory additives....

The way these dead animals wind up in your pet's food is through a process known as rendering.[41]

What Is "Rendering"?

The process of rendering begins with a mass of food animals (animals no longer living that will be recycled into meat for other animal consumption)—both whole animals and reject animal parts (such as heads, hooves, bones, offal [internal organs and entrails], blood, adipose tissue [fats], and cartilage, as well as cuts that fall into the "supermarket rejects" category, etc.)—that will ultimately serve as the meat and protein by-products in pet foods. (Note that these by-products are also used in many other marketed products, some intended for human use such as hygienic goods and cosmetics, but this book will not address those areas.) This mass is frequently referred to as "the raw." The raw is ground first with a large auger grinder, and then a second time into a finer, gooier mass with a smaller auger grinder. The raw is then cooked slowly, and the tallow (fat that rises to the top during the cooking process) is skimmed (or spun) from the top. The tallow is shipped off to be used in a variety of products (mostly soaps), and the remaining cooked meat by-products are sent to a hammer press, where the moisture is squeezed out completely. From there, it is run through a sifter to remove large gatherings of hair and leftover chippings of bone. The final remnants of the animals are finely ground to a powder.

Once the powder is complete and ready for shipping, it is purchased by major pet food companies as the ingredient for protein in their chow. (This is why, instead of seeing "chicken," "beef," or "pork" listed on many pet food labels, we see vague and misleading ingredients such as "meat by-product meal," "protein by-product meal," etc. [more on this later], which is generic, allowing almost anything to be mixed in a giant vat and ground into powder, as long as there was meat in it at some point, from some animal, somewhere. And, to the average consumers who merely want to make sure that Fido is getting his protein, this ingredient reassures them that the pros know what they're doing.)

Now that the rendered by-products are at the storage warehouse of the food manufacturing company cookhouses, they are added to the companies' pet food recipes, along with: preservatives to ensure a longer shelf life of the food; color dyes to appeal to the shopper's eye as well as to suggest that healthy vegetable ingredients are being used (orange kibbles suggest carrots, green kibbles suggest healthy greens, etc.); flavoring, often including ingredients like sugar that have utterly zero nutritional value for the pet and can cause behavioral problems (but result in an animal eating the food very quickly because it "tastes good," *not* because it is good for the animal…much like a child in a candy store); rice (and/or rice by-products, cereals, grains, etc.), corn; and a number of other ingredients, often including the minimal vitamin supplements required for the producer to be allowed to refer to the diet as a "specialized food" or "life-stage" food.

Concerns Regarding the Meat Sources Used?

Many concerns arise immediately regarding meat sources used in pet food, and many of those concerns would not be an issue if the meat included in pet foods came from reliable sources and not from a generic rendering plant. Though some suggest that all the horror stories surrounding the protein by-products produced at rendering plants are simply hearsay, some deeper research quickly confirms that some of these terrible practices are, in fact, happening all over the world.

Please note as you read: According to the FDA definition of "food" from Section 201 (f): "The term 'food' means (1) articles used for food or drink for man *or other animals*, (2) chewing gum, and (3) articles used for components of any such article."[42] And according to Section 402, subsection article 342 regarding "adulterated" foods: "A food shall be deemed to be adulterated—(a) Poisonous, insanitary, or deleterious ingredients…. [(a)(5)] if it is, in whole or in part, the product of a diseased animal or of an animal which has died otherwise than by slaughter."[43]

Let's visit some of these concerns.

Rotten, Old, Filthy Meat/*Dirty Jobs* Episode

Rendering plants are very secretive about their practices. If you call one and ask for a tour of their facilities, it is likely that you will face the same red tape as many other researchers. Simply put: Rendering plant operators *do not* want anyone seeing what goes into their grinders. If they were responsible and on the level about what goes on behind their factory doors, then what would they have to hide?

However, one brave fellow hailing from the North State Rendering plant in Oroville, California, decided to open up about his plant's procedures in a major way. Agreeing to participate in the Discovery Channel's *Dirty Jobs* television show, he welcomed host Mike Rowe and his camera crew to make a few observations.

(To the reader who has never heard of this show, each episode starts with an explanation of one or two jobs that qualify as "dirty." Then, host Rowe dons the appropriate apparel for the job and plows straight into the duties of a typical employee on the job, walking the viewer through the most unfathomable occupational experiences a person can imagine. He has wrestled alligators in mud pits, swum through sewage, collected road kill, cleaned chimneys, exterminated insects, synthetically inseminated farm animals, and worked with hordes of exotic animals in obscure maintenance settings [and the list goes on and on], as well as completed dangerous feats in the process. If there is a terrible, nasty job out there, Mike Rowe addressed it for eight seasons straight, with the series ending in 2012.)

The entire episode entitled "Animal Rendering" was unbelievably gross. And yet, because it was nationally broadcast on one of the world's most popular channels, one must assume that *this* is one of the cleaner rendering houses.

Only seven seconds into the program, a warning appears on screen to caution viewers that what they are about to see is graphic, disturbing, and for mature audiences only.[44] Following this, Rowe briefly explains the purpose of rendering as a part of farming culture (because the reader has already been educated about the purpose and system of rendering, we will not summarize his comments here). After explaining the purposes of recycling cows, Rowe tells the viewer, "The process is called rendering, and it's good for the environment, and the bottom line. And it's as bad as bad gets in every other way."[45]

He wasn't kidding.

As Rowe begins his day collecting dead cows with fellow deceased livestock collector Lupé, the camera pans over several dead cows left in a heap at the edge of a fence, with a fully operational farm in the background. The cows are literally so bloated, Rowe asks Lupé, "What are the odds of one of these things [cows] exploding?" Lupé responds, "Sometimes, they do."[46] The reason for the bloating is obvious: The animals have been left out in the sun to bake in the heat and a swarm of maggots for days. Flies are buzzing in a small, dark, busy cloud energetically whizzing about the carcasses.

After Rowe quips about the "job security" that Lupé has as a result of having a career nobody would ever want,[47] Lupé gestures to a swollen cow. "This one's been dead for like, four days," he says. Rowe kneels down, pointing. "Ohhh, just maggots, right?" he says. Sections of this filthy, long-dead cow have huge chunks of flesh missing from its udder; the camera takes a close-up of a part of the animal that is so covered in maggots that its hide cannot be seen underneath.[48]

But about the time the viewer is wondering what in the otherworld this recyclable "meat" could possibly be used for, Rowe narrates its purpose: "North State turns out millions of pounds of rendered product every year. The final result is used to manufacture hundreds of products. Everything from soap to candles to *pet food* to cosmetics."[49] Now, at the processing facility, the plant is filled with dead, maggoty cows all the way to the door, forcing Rowe to climb on top of and walk over the carcasses—grabbing dead body parts and flesh for leverage to steady himself—just to get inside. He looks at the camera with obvious disgust and says, "Rendering. What fresh hell is this?"[50]

The camera pans about and zooms in on the first arrival room. The concrete floor is wet with blood and something black that isn't identified (maybe it's just dirty water?). The back walls are insanely grimy, with big gouges and chipped paint, and plaster peeking through in spots. It's a perfect broken-down, abandoned-building setting for a Quentin Tarantino torture flick.

Rowe greets a man named Chris, who explains that his family has been in this business for going on four generations.

Then, for all the viewers wondering why in the world one of these plants would ever allow this kind of terrible exposure, Rowe says: "I called *everybody* looking for a place that could honestly show us what happens [at a rendering plant], because I know that this is an important part of the whole farming reality.... How come you're the only person who said 'yes' [to allowing the *Dirty Jobs* crew to come in and film their practice]?"

"I'm probably crazy," Chris responds with a chuckle, then hunkers down for an attempt at a real answer. "I don't know, but it's been a quiet industry, and you know, I think it's time people realize what we do. We recycle a lot of stuff, and we're a key part of the food chain. We really are."[51]

Chris proceeds to allow Rowe to fill a cow with air in order to separate the hide from the body, and then he finishes the skinning job with a knife, pulling the hide from the meat in the stubborn spots where the air didn't do the trick. Nobody attempts to clean the maggots from the cow before the commencement of this step, so, once again, the camera grabs a close-up of the wriggling as an inflation hole is cut for the air hose. During the skinning, Rowe inquires whether this specific rendering house sticks only to cows, or if they take in other animals. Chris gives a small list, including horses, llamas, and eggs, but the scene blips to another shot before he finishes the list.[52] When the cow is skinned, Rowe is instructed to drop the hide down a hole in the floor, a "chute" leading to the "cellar," where the hide is later salted for preservation and sold. The door of the chute is recognizable by a trail of blood leading away from the carcasses. At this point, Rowe and Chris share a brief, but enlightening, exchange:

ROWE: So this room, as bad as it is and as rough as it looks, is actually on top of another room.

CHRIS: That's correct.

ROWE: That I can only assume looks worse.

CHRIS: Yes.[53]

Following this, a conversation ensues regarding the fate of the "ingredients." It is mentioned that the product will go to feed other animals, and Chris specifically acknowledges that the "feed" powder will be available to "whoever buys it that wants to make [or use] it."[54] (Evidently, the rendering plants are not picky about whom they sell their powders to.)

The skinless cow is now connected to a chain and raised into the grinder. The entire cow is processed, from his head to his back hooves, until nothing remains on the hook.

ROWE: The bones, the organs, the intestines, the stomach, the liver, the meat, all of it, straight into the feed.

CHRIS: We waste nothing.[55]

Disturbingly, the camera does show where the cow comes out on the other end of the grinder: a huge holding hopper containing the grinds of this, and many other, entire animals.

(As a side note, many assume that dogs and cats will eat any part of the animal offered to them as food. These authors have heard this statement off and on throughout life, to the tune of, "Yeah, but a dog out there in the wild would eat the whole animal to survive. They don't care. Meat is meat." This not always true. An animal out in the wild will pick the flesh off the bone, and then chew the bone, but these "wild animals" will almost always leave behind organs, brains, intestines, etc.)

As viewers of the TV show break away from the arrival room, we are taken on a quick visual journey over giant vats and grinders where other meat and bones are being dumped by trucks. Rowe acknowledges their source: "North State also recycles truckloads of discarded meat [the "rejects"] from slaughterhouses, butcher shops, even restaurants."[56] The "meat" being poured into the grinder contains plastic bags and pieces of garbage. Nobody has bothered to sift through and remove these foreign objects from the protein sources. And for the viewers who may be thinking that perhaps these secondary meat sources end up in a different place for a purpose other than feed for animals, this simply is not the case, based on the following scene: Rowe stands at the top of the conveyor belts and shows that the plastic-bagged "stuff that guy in the truck dropped off" is coming up on one conveyor, and the other conveyor carrying the meat from the arrival room hopper are dumping into one slide, where they are then distributed straight into the cookers.[57]

In the cooking room, Rowe explains, "There are actually three cooking tanks in this building. Each one of them holds six and a half tons of [he pauses, then says sarcastically], oh, let's call them, 'ingredients.'"[58] The smell in the air is foul, as Rowe places his hand against his nose and mouth, and a few seconds later, says to his viewers, "I wish you could smell it!"[59] A moment later, the camera focuses in on Rowe as he asks Chris, "What's making my throat close up here?" Chris' response is a humorous comment that perhaps it's because Rowe is hungry.[60] It is during this time that the process of getting the tallow (Chris calls it "oil") to separate from the meat, and the meat being turned into powder, is explained.

Rowe, anxious to leave the room, follows Chris out.

The rest of this episode is focused on machine maintenance, the follow-up of the cellar containing the hides, and a few other things unrelated to the food product that will be shipped out to our pet's foods. For the sake of focus, we will end our commentary on this show now.

From this one video source alone—featuring one rendering plant owner so confident of his proper handling that he would allow the Discover Channel network to film it—we have evidence of the following:

- The meat source animals are dead for many days, left to bloat and rot in the hot sun before delivery to the rendering plants.
- Maggots and flies swarm around the carcasses, which are not cleaned before processing.
- Rendering plants are secretive and hide their practices behind red tape (as Rowe says in the beginning of the episode).
- The "raw" is handled and processed in extremely filthy and revolting conditions.
- It is confirmed that this rendering plant sells its

products to pet food companies as well as to "whoever" else wants it.

- "Rejects" including plastic bags and garbage from secondary sources are added to the "raw."

Let's continue.

Euthanized Pets? Hazardous Chemical Injections?

For some readers, the idea of a euthanized animal from a pet shelter being delivered to the rendering floor is shocking enough to inspire instant skepticism. We don't blame you. That was our reaction as well. But, Hersh Pendell, former AAFCO president, was featured in a news cover story regarding the pet food industry. The following is an excerpt from a news clip of that release:

NEWSCASTER: Pendell says he's not aware of any written law or regulation at *any* level, specifically prohibiting the use of rendered products, which contain dead cats and dogs....

PENDELL: [I]t may not be acceptable, but nutritionally, it's still protein.

NEWS CREWMAN: Can we tell what's in pet food just by looking at the label?

PENDELL: There's no way to really tell that, because

if the ingredient says "meat and bone meal," you don't know if that's cattle, or sheep, or horse, or "Fluffy" [referring to a pet's common domestic name].[61]

And there is no reason to believe that, other than "Fluffy," as Pendell so casually states, the rest of the meat used is even remotely clean, fresh, properly handled, or fit for healthy consumption by any living creature, as addressed in the previous section of this chapter. Though Chris only showed livestock in his plant, other eyewitness accounts include reports of dogs, cats, and other animals being taken to rendering plants. Heart-wrenching and nightmare-inducing stories circulate the media, books, articles, and the Internet, unabashedly containing testimonies from workers at these rendering plants as well as from visitors to these locations. One needs only to Google the subject to be inundated with uncountable credible sources citing this practice. Take, for example, the recollection of Keith Woods, in his article "The Dark Side of Recycling" for *Earth Island Journal*:

> The rendering plant floor is piled high with "raw product." Thousands of dead dogs and cats; heads and hooves from cattle, sheep, pigs and horses; whole skunks; rats and raccoons—all waiting to be processed.
>
> In the ninety-degree heat, the piles of dead animals seem to have a life of their own *as millions of maggots swarm over the carcasses*.
>
> Two bandanna-masked men begin operating Bobcat mini-dozers, loading the "raw" into a ten-foot deep stainless steel pit.[62]

Although the *Dirty Jobs* episode did *not* indicate that the meat was ever cleaned, other sources address this meat-cleaning process; however, it's not comforting.

The chemicals used to disinfect the meats can be extremely harmful if consumed. In another article called "Food Not Fit for a Pet," originally appearing in *Let's Live Magazine* (later quoted and published in full numerous times within several credible publications, including *Earth Island Journal*), Wendell Belfield, DVM, had this to say:

> For seven years, I was a veterinary meat inspector for the US Department of Agriculture and the State of California. I waded through blood, water, pus and fecal material, inhaled the fetid stench from the killing floor and listened to the death cries of slaughtered animals....
>
> To prevent condemned meat from being rerouted and used for human consumption, government regulations require that meat is "denatured" before removal from the slaughterhouse and shipment to rendering facilities. In my time as a veterinary meat inspector, we denatured with carbolic acid (a potentially corrosive disinfectant) and/or creosote (used for wood-preservation or as a disinfectant). Both substances are highly toxic. According to federal meat inspection regulations, fuel oil, kerosene, crude carbolic acid and citronella (an insect repellent...) all are approved denaturing materials.
>
> Condemned livestock carcasses treated with these

chemicals can become meat and bone meal for the pet food industry. Because rendering facilities are not government-controlled, any animal carcasses can be rendered—even dogs and cats. As Eileen Layne of the CVMA [California Veterinary Medical Association] told the Chronicle, "When you read pet food labels, and it says 'meat and bone meal,' that's what it is: cooked and converted animals, including some dogs and cats."

Some of these dead pets—those euthanised by veterinarians—already contain pentobarbital before treatment with the denaturing process. According to University of Minnesota researchers, the sodium pentobarbital used to euthanise pets "survives rendering without undergoing degradation." Fat stabilisers are introduced into the finished rendered product to prevent rancidity.[63]

What does "survives rendering without undergoing degradation" mean? Simply that the chemical that killed Pet A at the shelter or veterinary clinic when it was put to sleep has not been neutralized or cancelled out by the rendering process. Pet A's body is added to the "raw" and ground with the rest of the protein sources, where its poison is allowed to spread to, and affect, the other protein by-products in the cooker. After the rendering is over, the powder is sent to the manufacturers, and the new food is packaged and shelved at stores, Pet B will ingest a portion of the poison that killed Pet A. How *much* Pet B will receive of the euthanizing drug is anyone's guess, because the number of euthanized pets added to the raw in a single rendering batch varies in each case. However, we know that, as stated by the Humane Society, "About 2.4 million healthy, adoptable cats and dogs—about one every 13 seconds—are put down in U.S. shelters each year. Often these animals are the [unintended] offspring of cherished family pets."[64]

Close your eyes. Count to thirteen. A "healthy, adoptable" cat or dog was just put to death, because some months ago Fido got loose or Fluffy was in heat and conceived an unwanted litter. This doesn't even count the "unhealthy, diseased" cat or dog that was put down because of a physical malady destroying their body from the inside out (which, as you will read later, could be up to another twelve million, including animals humanely euthanized at late stages of cancer). That's a *lot* of euthanized pet animals per year whose physical remains require a resting place of some sort. Some veterinary clinics offer to cremate animals, but this is often at an added expense. Some cities allow pet owners to take the remains home for burial. Other disposal strategies when veterinary staff (or shelters) become desperate have heralded several shocking headlines over the years, such as, "NYC Veterinarian Charged with Dumping 35 Euthanized Cats, Dogs, and Lizard Alongside Highway."[65] This is only one article by the Associated Press representing uncountable others that we will never hear about because nobody was ever caught in the act. Needless to say, there is a very real and ever-present need for shelters and clinics to dispose of pet remains. And, all the while, the rendering companies are looking for the quickest, cheapest meat sources to add to their eerie brew of protein by-products, so we can be sure it's not hard to find a pick-up service willing to haul away the remains for a trip to the rendering plant at no charge to the shelter or clinic. It's not hard to imagine that shelters and clinics would find releasing the remains to a rendering facility mutually beneficial.

A video called *What's REALLY in Your Pet's FOOD??* captured by an investigator for the Campaigns Department of LCA (Last Chance for Animals), based in Beverly Hills, California, is circulating the Internet right now. The video begins by featuring a rendering company, the D & D Disposal West Coast Rendering in Vernon, California, in 2007, and it shows the following (these authors *highly* advise any reader with a squeamish stomach or close bond to a pet *not* to watch this incredibly disturbing video):

- Euthanized pet animals are taken from a veterinary clinic freezer in plastic bags.
- Pets' whole-body remains are placed in barrels and bags; some are recognizable without any external wrapping/covering.
- The camera closes in on a collection of barrels, the sheer number of which—each containing the frozen bodies of domestic household pets—is astounding.
- The euthanized pets are then taken and unloaded into what the video refers as "the pit" at the D & D Disposal West Coast Rendering facility.
- The animals are put through the grinder.
- The cookers are shown processing the meal.
- And finally, the end product—protein by-product meal powder—is shown.[66]

Some of the comments under this posting (many of which involve profanity, just as a warning to the readers) reflect feedback suggesting that this video doesn't prove anything because it's merely poor-quality, muted video clips that someone later on layered with text. The video can't prove that the rendering plant listed at the beginning of the video is the actual plant being filmed on the tape, *or* that the end product is going into your pet's food. There is also no named investigator willing to stand up and claim the footage, or give any eyewitness testimony of exactly what he or she saw. The various clips could have been taken from several different locations and edited together as a falsified scare tactic.

That could be anyone wanting to stir up controversy, correct? Sure.

So, these authors dug a little deeper, to see if this obscure online video had any clout to its claims.

To begin, a call was placed to the LCA in Beverly Hills, in hopes that they would, in fact, acknowledge the video to be their own. This at a minimum would prove that the LCA publicly stands behind this as a legitimate investigation, and that their official position was that this video was not edited in any way to create an abstract, falsified series of claims about the rendering plant or the euthanized animals depicted. Within the hour, Karen from the campaigns department of LCA returned the call. It took a minute or two to direct her to the video in question, and she recognized it immediately. "Oh yes, this is definitely one of ours," she said. "Rendering is such a secretive business, and especially when it comes to euthanized animals and improper meat sources." Within one minute, she helped us find that video embedded within their own website on a page with more information about the investigation they launched in May of 2007. Within this page, the uses for the "raw" in question were listed, and the first two items on the list were "livestock feed" and "pet foods and treats."[67] (The video was also uploaded to YouTube in 2009, about a year after the other one mentioned, which may explain the fewer number of views.[68])

When asked whether this kind of practice was still occurring, Karen said, "LCA has not, as an organization, investigated this for a while, but there is certainly no reason to believe that this has been stopped, because it's all perfectly legal. In order for this practice to be stopped, there has to be a lot of awareness and laws preventing it, and we're just not there yet. In the meantime, nobody in the rendering business will open up about it. Everyone is very secretive."

She was unable to divulge the identity of the investigator for privacy purposes.

As it turns out, a report was conducted in 2004 by the County of Los Angeles Department of Animal Care and Control involving the claims regarding D & D Disposal West Coast Rendering facility. That report birthed an article by *Contra Costa Times News* called "Firm Gives Remains of Euthanized Pets Another Use," which related the following:

> "Unfortunately, for government agencies, this is the most cost-effective option that's available and it's my understanding that's why every other agency uses this service," he [Brian Cronin, division chief for

San Bernardino County's Animal Care and Control Division] said....

Bill Gorman, president of D&D Disposal, said the firm doesn't conduct media interviews and declined to discuss what his company does with animal remains [big surprise].

But the April 2004 report by Los Angeles County Animal Shelters detailed how euthanized animals are · recycled in a process known as "rendering."... [69]

Earlier in the article, this subject caused concern for one coordinator with the Humane Society, who said, "As a Humane Society, we would never consent to allowing the bodies of these precious animals (to be) used in research or any medical uses and research, or certainly not to be re-used in a form of food for any purpose." So there is plenty of proof that the "good folks" out there would never allow this if they knew about it. Nonetheless, it appears that it *is* happening, and there appears to be proof upon just a little digging.

Naturally, our next phone call was to the City of San Bernardino Animal Control facility, since it was listed in the article as having tended to "13,396" euthanized animals the previous year, and was said to send those animals to D & D Disposal West Coast Rendering. If this were confirmed, it would be another link to proving that what was said in this disturbing video was factual. The very first person we encountered on this phone call—a receptionist named Abda—was kind and helpful. We asked, "Once the animals are euthanized in your shelter, what happens to them from there?" Her response confirmed that things had recently changed, but that "a few years ago" (including the time this video was shot), they had a contract with D & D. We continued the conversation to a conclusion we saw from a mile away:

DONNA HOWELL: Once D & D took the animals, what did they do with them? We've heard they rendered them into pet foods.

ABDA: Uh-huh. [There was not an ounce of shock in her voice.]

DONNA HOWELL: Is that true, then? Is that what they do with them?

ABDA: I honestly can't say. You would have to call and ask them [D & D].

Now, not only is it a sure deal that the video was a legitimate filming from an undercover LCA investigator, but it was now also confirmed that one of the largest animal shelters in the country had a contract with D & D to retrieve the euthanized animals and take them to a rendering plant at the time the video was shot. What caused the City of San Bernardino Animal Control facility to change its practice of sending their euthanized animals to D & D? It's only a guess, but it may be because of all the media related to the LCA investigation, as well as the report written up by Los Angeles County Department of Animal Care and Control.

But shelters are not the same as veterinary clinics, so we looked into that as well. The San Diego County website released a document from the "Office of the County Veterinarian" called "Options for Animal Disposal." This document reveals that:

> The following options are available for disposal of deceased [euthanized] animals:
> - Onsite burial
> - Cremation/Cemeteries
> - Landfills
> - Private companies[70]

Upon scrolling to the bottom of the document, under the "Private Companies" subhead, the very first company listed was D & D.

By now, the reader is likely wondering if we ever questioned D & D directly. We did. Our first phone call *did* confirm that D & D Disposal is the same company as West Coast Rendering. We ended up speaking with a somewhat nervous voice on the other end of the line—the voice of a person who would not give us a name:

D & D: D & D, how can I help you?

DONNA HOWELL: Oh, I may have the wrong number. I was trying to get in touch with West Coast Rendering Services?

D & D: Yes, go ahead. How can we help you?

DONNA HOWELL: I'm just curious. I've heard that D & D picks up animals from all the surrounding shelters. Is that correct?

D & D: No, we don't euthanize animals here.

DONNA HOWELL: But the shelters and veterinary clinics do.

D & D: Uhhh, yes.

DONNA HOWELL: And D & D picks them up?

D & D: Yes, yes we do.

DONNA HOWELL: And once you have picked them up, where do they go?

D & D: We render them.

DONNA HOWELL: And by rendering, you mean they are turned into protein by-products, correct?

D & D: Yes.

DONNA HOWELL: Who are these by-products sold to? What products come from them?

D & D: I'm not sure I know what you mean.

DONNA HOWELL: The protein by-products. The end product when these euthanized animals are rendered. Where does that go? [Silence on the other end.] Is that powder turned into soaps? Or animal feed? Or?

D & D: One moment. Let me get you to someone who can help you.

DONNA HOWELL: Thank you, and what was your name?

D & D: Yes, one moment.

That was a puzzling answer to a simple question like "What was your name?"—especially when the person on the other line did not have an accent, and did not give any reason to believe there was a language barrier… Nonetheless, we remained on hold for a minute, and the call went dead.

No problem. It happens. Lines disconnect. We called back. After re-explaining ourselves to the same person, and once again asking what the rendered powder gets turn into, we were asked:

D & D: Where are you calling from?

DONNA HOWELL: Missouri.

D & D: What *company* are you calling from?

DONNA HOWELL: You mean who do I work for?

D & D: Yes, what company is asking these things?

DONNA HOWELL: [On the spot, all that could be said was the truth.] I'm calling from a publishing company, and I am looking to gain some insight into the practices of rendering houses for a project we are working on.

D & D: I see. Please hold.

This time, we were not given the opportunity to ask for a name. We were on hold for a couple of minutes when another, more upbeat, voice came on the line. She introduced herself as Christina. She was kind and pleasant.

CHRISTINA: This is Christina. How may I help you?

DONNA HOWELL: Hello, I called a few minutes ago and had a few questions regarding your rendered by-products.

CHRISTINA: Yes, they told me. What specific questions can I answer for you?

DONNA HOWELL: I heard that your company picks up euthanized animals from shelters and veterinary clinics. Is that correct?

CHRISTINA: Uh-huh. All over the area. Yep.

DONNA HOWELL: I also heard that you render these euthanized animals. Is that also correct?

CHRISTINA: Yep.

DONNA HOWELL: I do have one concern. I am reading information in my research that suggests that your protein by-products are sent to pet food companies, meaning that the euthanized animals are being recycled into our domestic pet foods. Is this true?

CHRISTINA: The by-products are sold to companies internationally. The company then decides what to use it for.

DONNA HOWELL: Internationally where?

CHRISTINA: To countries like China.

DONNA HOWELL: What do they use it for?

CHRISTINA: We are told to say that the by-products are used for things like fertilizer.

DONNA HOWELL: You are "told to say"?

CHRISTINA: Yes, they tell us to say that it's going to things like fertilizer.

DONNA HOWELL: Oh. Well, please know that this next

question is given with complete respect, but if it's being shipped to countries like China, and you are being told what to say, how do you know what they are really doing with it?

CHRISTINA: That's true. We really don't know. We just ship it. If they are making pet food out of it, then that's not our [she pauses]… I guess we don't always know exactly. They just tell us to say they are making things like fertilizer out of it. That's really all I can tell you.

DONNA HOWELL: I see. Well, it's not your fault that they don't give you complete disclosure, I guess.

CHRISTINA: Right. [She chuckles.]

DONNA HOWELL: And this "they" that you are referring to. Any chance you can tell me who this "they" is that you're sending the by-products to? What companies are on that list?

CHRISTINA: No, I'm sorry. I'm not allowed to say. That's confidential information.

With that, we thanked her sincerely for her time and let her get back to her job. At the onset, the idea that we were at least getting an answer about where the products were going, and that they were focusing on fertilizer, was encouraging. On the other hand, there was a substantial lack of information offered during both phone calls, and the first person we spoke to sounded nervous that we were asking. We were not allowed to speak with Christina until after we had stated that we worked in the media—and of course, that automatically delivers biased answers when one knows he or she is may be quoted in a publication. We are not allowed to know who these companies are, or what *exactly* they do with the by-products. Christina could *not* confirm that the by-products were not going into pet foods. She could—and *did*—confirm that she had been given specific instructions as to what to say when someone calls.

For anyone still in doubt over D & D, we will admit that there is still no irrefutable evidence that places euthanized animal remains in Fido's bowl where *that specific* rendering company is concerned. However, remember that it was a number of years ago when D & D's name was dragged through the mud regarding the end location and purpose of their products, so they would have a lot of reasons to steer clear of associating with pet foods by the year 2015. Additionally, assuming the operators of the plant are completely innocent now, that doesn't mean they were innocent in 2007 during the time of the LCA investigation.

We have only used *one* rendering plant as an example of whether euthanized animals are recycled into pet foods. There are many more out there. Based on this phone call, sometimes not even the employees of the plant, themselves, know where the end product is going. We can bet that if a pet food company out there can get hold of some cheap by-products, they are going to use it.

Still, some may doubt that this could possibly be true. It all sounds just too hard to believe. If there isn't any irrefutable truth to this D & D story, is there at least proof somewhere else that this is happening?

After investigating the subject from the red-tape angle, these authors saw another avenue worth exploring. Jenny Lynn, veteran kennel operator and former assistant to several humane societies and animal control centers in the state of Missouri and Illinois, agreed to an exclusive, personal interview on the subject of euthanized pets and the possibility of their remains being rendered into protein powder for inclusion in future pet foods. The following is an excerpt from that conversation:

JOE ARDIS: Which state were you an assistant for dog kennels and animal control facilities?

JENNY LYNN: Illinois, and in the Taney, Greene, and Stone counties of Missouri. I worked at several different kennels and facilities.

JOE ARDIS: What were some of your job descriptions during that time?

JENNY LYNN: I took care of the dogs and other animals. I did tons of cleaning, bathing, and clipping dogs. Each place I worked at was different. In Illinois, I worked for animal control and did all the nasty jobs, including tying up all the dogs so my lead officer could go through and euthanize them. Some dogs [took a long time to pass away after injection] and he would [deliver a death blow] if the euthanasia didn't kill them. I just remember their eyes. That will haunt me forever.

I also volunteered at several humane societies, and I worked at four different kennels in Missouri. One of them was actually really nice and could have been a model for all dog breeders to follow!

JOE ARDIS: In the places that you worked, what were some of the ways they would dispose of the euthanized animals' remains?

JENNY LYNN: One place dug a pit with a backhoe and buried them. One place threw the remains in the "lagoon," Missouri's version of a septic system. Each place took care of the remains of dead animals differently, but…it was usually pretty crude. One humane society in Missouri had a rendering plant pick up the remains, which were sent to a mill to be ground up and processed into dog and cat food, as well as some other feeds like chicken and hog feed.[71]

And with validation from an inside source such as this, the only thread that seemingly remains loose is proof from a source that *anyone* can access: the government.

Despite the FDA's assertion that the "levels of exposure to sodium pentobarbital (pentobarbital) [the drugs used to euthanize an animal] that dogs might receive through food is unlikely to cause them any adverse health effects," they openly acknowledge that rendering plants take in animal remains containing the fatal drug. Directly from the FDA website:

Because in addition to producing anesthesia, pentobarbital is routinely used to euthanize animals, the most likely way it could get into dog food would be in rendered animal products.

Rendered products come from a process that converts animal tissues to feed ingredients. Pentobarbital seems to be able to survive the rendering process. If animals are euthanized with pentobarbital and subsequently rendered, pentobarbital could be present in the rendered feed ingredients.[72]

The FDA is not in any hurry to do anything *about* it, but there it is: an acknowledgement of the practice straight from the horse's mouth. And the idea that the "levels of exposure" are "unlikely to cause [your pet] any adverse health effects" is largely up for debate. If a pet were to be given a food with this ingredient once or twice, I'm sure this statement would be true. But two or three times a day for the extent of the pet's life of feeding on cheap commercial foods? It's not rocket science.

Additionally, one may notice that this report contains notes regarding the presence of the pentobarbital as belonging to euthanized cattle or horses, because the feed did not produce any DNA evidence of cats and dogs within the feed. If this were true, wouldn't that prove that euthanized domestic dogs and cats were not involved in this particular render batch? Not exactly.

Extreme heat, such as that which would be applied to the food animals during the rendering process, likely destroys all DNA evidence. Also note that the tests were completed on commercial kibble, already dried and bagged (and therefore several manufacturing steps beyond the rendering plant itself, suggesting with near certainty that the render powder was heated a second time during the formation of the kibble bits, for double the heat exposure).

We asked Sharon Gilbert—author of *The Armageddon Strain*, whose formal education includes theology, molecular biology, and genetics—if she thought DNA would survive the rendering process and therefore be detectable in post-rendered "meal." Her answer was enlightening. "DNA is a very delicate molecule. It is true that DNA is destroyed when it is exposed to extreme heat. If the rendering plant in question had, in fact, applied high degrees of heat during the rendering process, then it is highly likely that the DNA from any cat or dog would be destroyed and, therefore, be undetectable in subsequent DNA testing of the animal feed." This opinion was also reflected by Peter Faletra, PhD, as quoted in Ann Martin's *Food Pets Die For*. However, Gilbert went on to say:

> I did a little sleuthing for the most recent updates in the literature about DNA surviving high heat, and apparently some does survive even temperatures of 300-400 Kelvin if the molecule is "protected" by resistant tissues such as teeth, bone, and some fats. Also, the effect of high heat is to "unzip" the double stranded molecule, but depending on how long the material is heated and how quickly it cools, the molecule can sometimes re-anneal (go back together). This process forms the scientific basis of modern PCR detection methods. Because some DNA does occasionally sur-

vive, food inspectors have been able to detect horse DNA in dog food (when the meat source is labeled as other than horse, eg. buffalo, chicken, lamb). So, if you're looking to detect dog DNA (and dogs are often rendered at plants), then it might be possible.

It should also be noted that as our technology surrounding the testing of DNA improves, more and more, we can spot it where we would not have been able to prior. This particular test, done years ago, likely would not have showed elements of dog or cat DNA.

Martin, leaving no stone unturned, contacted the director of the Henry C. Lee Institute of Forensic Science, Dr. Albert Harper, for comment. Harper confirmed to Martin that it's "highly unlikely" that any DNA would be "identifiable" after the prolonged exposure to the kinds of cooking methods associated with pet food manufacturing.[73]

So, whether D & D is behind it, or whether the companies in China that claim to be making "fertilizer" are behind it, we know that pentobarbital is getting into the food. Of that, there is proof. Of the idea that the pentobarbital originated from a food animal source such as a euthanized pet dog or cat taken from a shelter or clinic, we also have a very likely scenario, *regardless* of whether "tests" prove the already-destroyed and therefore undetectable DNA is not present.

And before we assume that it is only dogs and cats, understand that a vast population of other animals from the farming community is also euthanized per year (cattle, horses, sheep, goats, and on and on), each of whose remains are even more likely to end up at a rendering plant, merely because of their association as food sources to begin with and not as "pets." There would be much less a risk of controversy if the public hears that a rendering plant may recycle a cow, rather than an animal regarded with a heightened status to humans, such as "member of the family," as many pets are. There may be no limit to the number of animals that have expired due to fatal drugs coursing through their veins—finding a free ride to a rendering plant where they will unconsciously poison the food of future animals.

But, is there proof that the practice of allowing Pentobarbital into pet foods will actually harm my animal?

Is your animal one of many that has died prematurely from unnatural causes? Has your pet been, like *uncountable* others, sick for some unknown reason, then suddenly showed new vibrancy when given a healthier diet? Is your animal starting to show symptoms of a dry coat, itchy spots, saggy eyelids, obesity, or a lack of energy?

Will second-hand poisoning sessions—a fatal drug ingested in small doses, several times a day, every day, over a long period of time—cause a number of health problems in your pet? Will rotten meat, *fuel oil, kerosene,* crude carbolic acid, creosote, insect repellant, and toxic, hazardous, corrosive disinfectants fed to your pet every day cause tumors and disease? Is there anyone out there who would doubt this connection?

According to the Animal Cancer Foundation, "roughly 6 million new cancer diagnoses are made in dogs and a similar number made in cats each year."[74] That's six million dogs plus an approximate six million cats per year, equaling *twelve million* cases of cancer in one calendar year *in the US alone*! Perhaps not each diagnosis is a result of slow poisoning from a diet, but how many animals could have fared better had healthier foods been available? This is not even counting the deaths resulting from non-cancer related diseases/conditions, which we have a lot of reason to believe can also stem from the slow poisoning within a bad diet, leading to lower immunities, generally poorer health, and ripe targets for more diseases/conditions as their systems break down.

It's just a cycle that goes on and on: Pets get sick from bad food, they die, and they are recycled into bad food.

Not surprisingly, feeding a dog or cat with the meat from another animal that was chemically euthanized ultimately does not lead to a healthy, balanced diet. A long, vigorous life is not the outcome of one fed diseased zoo or farm animals.

It's common sense.

And yet, the action that common sense would naturally produce—the discontinuation of this practice within the manufacturing of pet foods—is typically inhibited by the lack of public awareness and therefore any potential action against it. It's a standard, wool-over-the-eyes, hush-hush, cloak-and-dagger (you've heard them all) covert functioning of the pet food industry, driven by greedy money-mongrels to save a buck on meat sources. If this was still a well-kept secret, then even the authors of this book would chalk all this up to conspiratorial nonsense. Yet, sadly, the truth is out, and has been out for years. Even the *Dogs Naturally Magazine* quote above referred to it as "old news for many."However, because of brilliant ad schemes with convincing lingo about "science" and "research" and picturing men in lab coats, the wool remains over the eyes of the vast majority of pet owners.

Road Kill? Plastic? Styrofoam? ID Tags?

By now, the reader is likely willing to accept that there are confirmed cases of terrible things going on in the pet food industry. Could these money-mongers also be placing *road kill* into the mix?

Robert Hadnot, a "refuge collection truck operator" (fancy words for "road kill collector") in Los Angeles, was picking up dead animals from the road for the city's Sanitation Department of Public Works. The animals were maggot-riddled, in ditches, half-eaten, or decomposed (just as you would expect any animal lying around in the sun for days on end to be). Often, Hadnot gets a phone call with a specific address where a domestic pet animal has expired at home. Those must be disposed of as well. For Hadnot, retrieving deceased animals is a daily part of living in the great, sunny state of California.

In a recent video, Hadnot explains, "It's just too many animals on the streets, and they wind up getting hit. They have no homes to go to. They're not fed. So, this is the thing that happens."[75]

Richard Mayer, division manager of the valley collection area for the Bureau of Sanitation of the city of Los Angeles, works alongside good people like the compassionate Hadnot.

MAYER: The volume is about a hundred and twenty dead animals collected a day throughout the city. It starts out by getting a call from either a resident or a motorist… Sometimes a pet owner will call us and say it's expired at home. We'll come by, by appointment, and pick the animal up. So, once they call us, it's a priority call for us, because of health reasons. We'll go out there and pick him up.

OFF-CAMERA INTERVIEWER: And what happens to the dead animals?

MAYER: Once we collect it, uh, during the day, as the driver is out in the field, he'll go out with a load [containing] a sufficient quantity of animals, then they're taken to a rendering plant. There's a contractor that we work [with] that will render the animals.[76]

Although the pet food industry denies this (and they have every reason to if they want to stay in business), many, *many* sources confirm that this is a reality (including the reputable Dog Food Advisor online,[77] Truth about Pet Food,[78] and Ann Martin). According to the *LA Times*, "[S]ome [rendering] plants also mix in *road kill*, the trimmings from supermarket delis, dead farm animals and euthanized pets from shelters. Los Angeles city and county shelters send more than 120,000 dead dogs and cats to be rendered in a typical year."[79]

One authoritative source that at least acknowledges a category of protein in rendering plants referred to as "fallen animals" is the National Renderers Association. In its February 2009 "Buyer's Guide to Rendered Fats," it refers to "raw materials from various sources [including "fallen animals"]." Raw materials from *various* sources? To begin, the idea that "various sources" is the lingo opens up a Pandora's box of possibilities. Lynn Stratton of Healthy Holistic Living says this regarding the "fallen animals":

> It's the "fallen animals" part that seems extraordinarily open to interpretation, and again, note the use of the word "animals," not specific species, and "fallen," which doesn't exactly say how they fell. In fact, it's worth knowing that there are two categories of renderers, those actually attached to meat packing or food production facilities, and the ones known as independent renderers. The independents are the folks who pick up dead animals and their scraps, whether they're from your local supermarket or restaurant or from your local animal shelter or the side of the road. Then those truckloads are delivered to rendering plants, where the whole mess is boiled down into the euphemistically named "meat and bone meal" that winds up in your pet's food.
>
> And that also explains why your pet's food can contain such things as bits of ID tags, flea collars, antibiotic tags from livestock, and even plastic. The "Buyer's Guide to Rendered Fats" also notes that almost all tallow (a fat byproduct of the rendering process)

"contains polyethylene (PE), which is a foreign material in tallow, to some degree. It finds its way into the rendering plant as meat wrappers mixed in with the raw material. [Recall the part of the *Dirty Jobs* episode spoken of previously in this chapter: Anyone watching this on the Discovery Channel can stand as an eyewitness that plastic bags and garbage are being dumped into the hopper for inclusion in the grind.] Most of the polyethylene wrappers used by the meat industry are of low density type that will melt at lower temperatures and stay soluble in the tallow."

But how do meat wrappers get into your pet's food? When the truck heading to the rendering plant dumps its load of meat rejects from your local supermarket, including trimmings, refuse, offal (as bad as it sounds), and outdated packages of meat, they don't bother to remove the packaging. Think about that for a moment: The Styrofoam trays and the plastic wrap go right into the cooker with everything else.[80]

Additionally, there appears to be some acknowledgment from the FDA. According to their definition of "food" (mentioned early in this chapter): "The term 'food' means (1) articles used for food or drink for man *or other animals.*"[81] Again, regarding "adulterated" foods: "A food shall be deemed to be adulterated—(a) Poisonous, insanitary, or deleterious ingredients.... if it is, in whole or in part, the product of a diseased animal or of an animal which has died otherwise than by slaughter."[82] This appears to involve "fallen" animals, correct? But see the FDA CPG (Compliancy Guidance Manual) Section 675.400 "Rendered Animal Feed Ingredients" policy, which states: "*No regulatory action will be considered for animal feed ingredients resulting from the ordinary rendering process of industry, including those using animals which have died otherwise than by slaughter*, provided they are not otherwise in violation of the law."[83] Here we are told that these "fallen" animals that have "died otherwise than by slaughter" are okay to render and include in foods, as long as they are "not...in violation of the law." But rendering maggoty cows that have been dead for days at the edge of farms waiting for pickup by the rendering trucks is not in violation of the law. Would there be any difference between that cow and the deer someone hit on the highway days ago that is also bloated and riddled with maggots?

Conclusion

For readers who are still unconvinced, see the following, from the FDA's statement in the CPG under the heading, "CPG Section 690.500 Uncooked Meat for Animal Food":

BACKGROUND: *CVM [Center for Veterinary Medicine] is aware of the sale of dead, dying, disabled, or diseased (4-D) animals to salvagers for use as animal food.... The raw, frozen meat is shipped for use by several industries, *including pet food manufacturers* [!!!], zoos, greyhound kennels, and mink ranches. This meat *may present a potential health hazard to the animals that consume it* [!!!] and to the people who handle it.*

POLICY: *Uncooked meat derived from 4-D animals is adulterated under Section 402(a)(5) of the Act, and its shipment in interstate commerce for animal food use is subject to appropriate regulatory action.*[84]

Whew. For a second there, these authors thought there would be no "appropriate regulatory action." Thank goodness there was someone out there with our pets' best interest—

Oh, hang on a sec. The FDA page goes on to say:

REGULATORY ACTION GUIDANCE: *Districts should conduct preliminary investigations *only as follow-up to complaints or reports of injuries and should contact CVM before expending substantial resources.*[85]

Appropriate regulatory action takes place *only* as a follow up to complaints, because CVM can't expend substantial resources otherwise. What does this tell us? All pet owners with sick and dying pets should have their own resources— lots of money, lots of time, and the willingness to establish lots of veterinary paper trails since the beginning of the pet's illness symptoms, as mentioned earlier. Otherwise, we may be in trouble.

At the end of the day, it boils down to this: What the food animal rendering business isn't telling you *is* hurting your pet. If it has nothing to hide, then we would have more information and less red tape and hushed whispers. All the research in the world, all the finger-pointing and inquiries, won't prove anything as long as regulations aren't present and rendering plants aren't required to disclose information. But as long as they are not willing to disclose information, we can safely assume there is a reason for their unwillingness to tell us exactly what they are doing.

Why take the risk?

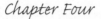

Chapter Four

Grains, Pains, and Other Things

While this may come as a surprise to you, commercial diets
are not well-suited to the dog's and cat's nutritional needs,
physical make up or metabolism. In other words, they simply,
are not "biologically appropriate." They are primarily made up
of grain products and are cooked/processed at high enough
temperatures to destroy any true available nutrition.
—The Whole Dog[86]

Protein is hugely important to our pets. Most pet owners and consumers know this already. Surprisingly, our nation continues to throw out exorbitant amounts of money on pet foods that list "corn" (or some nonprotein equivalent) as the first ingredient on the label. These pet foods are often the lowest-cost pet foods in stores, but they are frequently some of the most expensive, most attractive, and most misleading foods as well. Often, foods that are "veterinary recommended," "complete," or "balanced" don't list the protein sources within the ingredients until farther down the list—*after* all the grains and grain by-products that your pet either cannot digest or has a hard time digesting.

A few things need to be noted regarding the grains in pet foods, and we will discuss these at a greater length within this chapter. However, perhaps the most important place to start is the grains (and other related ingredients) associated with GMO practice.

Genetically Modified Organisms (GMO)

The world is becoming more and more aware of GMO foods and their effects within human biology. However, very few people seem to stop in their tracks to consider the consequences of GMO pet foods on our furry friends, *even though* the majority of scientific evidence gathered has primarily delivered documentation of the effects upon the animal kingdom.

What is GMO? As noted in the above heading, it stands for "genetically modified organisms." GMO is the process in which the genetic material (or genes) from one species is extracted and infused into the genes of a plant or animal with a completely separate genetic makeup. The purpose of this varies, but as an example, a GMO crop may be genetically engineered to hold more nutrients or to build up a higher resistance to insects, etc.

Initially, this sounds like a great idea. Why not borrow from one species to enhance another in order to develop super-plants with more nutrients and higher resistance to pests?

Unfortunately, the issue is really not that simple.

Monsanto, the highly controversial agrochemical corporation with specialization in agricultural biotechnology, remains the leading producer of GE (genetically engineered) seeds, as well as the developer behind Roundup, the top-selling herbicide (weed killer; pesticide) in the nation. (Note that this pesticide cannot be washed off.) Farmers rely heavily on Roundup to keep weeds at bay in their crops. The term "Roundup-ready crops" refers to crops that have been genetically modified to resist Roundup. The Roundup-ready crops have an advantage over standard crops because they will continue to thrive when sprayed near the unwanted foliage within a farm. However, glyphosate, the active ingredient in Roundup, is not safe for consumption, and this is obvious by the hazards listed on the warning label. It doesn't, however, keep the farming community from using it.

Surprisingly, however, issues surrounding the GMO controversy spread well beyond just the concerns regarding Roundup.

In the September 19, 2012, issue of the scientific journal, *Food and Chemical Toxicology*:

> [A]bout 200 albino Sprague-Dawley rats were divided into groups of 10 and fed diets with GM corn cultivated with or without the Roundup weed killer, or they were assigned to drink Roundup alone in water. Twenty rats served as controls.
>
> Female mice on GM diets were found to be two to three times more likely to die than those in the control group, and their health seemed to be more negatively affected by the diets whether it was sprayed with Roundup or not. About 50 percent of males and

70 percent of the females eating Monsanto GM corn died prematurely, compared to 30 percent of males and 20 percent of females not eating the corn.

Large mammary tumors developed in female rats about four months into the two-year study, some that were so large they blocked organ function.[87]

The science journal report caused a major stir, then was formally retracted when it came under pressure from large corporation-owned scientists. But the results of the study speak for themselves. Strangely, the report was *republished* a short time later in another science journal, proving that the interest of the health of the public, and not that of the corporations, was at least in this case superseding whether scientific evaluation should be hidden as a result of pressure from the powers that be.

Clearly based on this research, premature death, tumors, and negative health impacts are the result of ingesting ingredients obtained from GMO crops. In addition, the American Academy of Environmental Medicine "has raised a warning, based on some animal studies that GMO food consumption could be linked to health risks like infertility, immune disorders, insulin regulation, and more."[88] Other research has "linked GMOs to allergies, organ toxicity, and other serious health issues" within both animals and humans.[89] But those are not the only concerns. The research is still somewhat in the infancy years of development, since most GMO-related practice has become normative only recently, and even less-encouraging facts are available regarding the longer-term effects.

In a previous work of Thomas Horn on the "coming replacement humans" (*Forbidden Gates*, a book dedicated to the perilous implications of transhumanistic science upon our current and future generations), we read:

We have cited laboratory results in the past that were first reported by Dr. Árpád Pusztai, repeat verified by scientist Irina Ermakova, and later substantiated by the *International Journal of Biological Sciences* that showed genetically modified (GM) food had surprisingly ill effects on the health of test rats, including the deterioration of every animal organ, atrophied livers, altered cells, testicular damage, altered sperm counts, shortened life spans, and cancer development. The laboratory findings led to the biotech industry suppressing the data and an eight-year court battle with monster corporations that did not want these results made public.

Over the last several years, the silenced information has been in the news again as Greenpeace activists published evidence from the Russian trials verifying the ramifications of the negative health issues related to genetically modified foods. The wider ramifications from these and similar controlled experiments suggest that as current technology inserts pesticides, insect genes, animal DNA, and other modified organisms directly into crops, the threat of hybrid viruses, prion contamination and new disease strains—which humankind can neither anticipate or prepare for—

may arise. The prospects of this having an impact on mammalian health is almost certain to be a "when," not "if," concern, because, as Momma always said, "you are what you eat," and the fact that the food you consumed this week most likely contained genetically modified ingredients is a current reality.

For example, a large portion of the soybean, corn, cottonseed, and canola in today's human food supply and sold in most developed countries including the United States now has genes spliced in from foreign species—including bacteria and viruses—in its genetic makeup. These genetically modified organisms have not only been linked to sickness, sterility, allergies, and even death among *animals*, but the Institute for Responsible Technology (IRT) documents how the functioning genetically modified genes from these foods linger inside the human body, which could be future-catastrophic. "The only published human feeding experiment verified that genetic material inserted into GM soy transfers into the DNA of intestinal bacteria and continues to function," IRT published. "This means that long after we stop eating GM foods, we may still have their GM proteins produced continuously inside us."

Among other things, IRT says this means that: 1) If the antibiotic gene inserted into most GM crops were to transfer, it could create super diseases resistant to antibiotics; 2) If the gene that creates Bt toxin in GM corn were to transfer, it might turn our intestinal flora into living pesticide factories; and 3) Animal studies show that DNA in food can travel into organs throughout the body, even into the fetus.... Due to the large corporations (that stand to make billions of dollars from these products) having co-opted the FDA into not requiring food labeling or package warnings on GMO foods and health products, you and I are now the biggest lab rats of all time in a "wait-and-see" experiment that will, feasibly within the decade, illustrate whether Pusztai and Ermakova's rodent findings apply to us and our children.[90]

Horn is, of course, raising an argument about the long-term effects of GMO foods within the human diet. However, GMO foods may be harming our pets as much or even more than they are harming us. To begin, "genetically engineered corn made up 85 percent of acreage in 2013."[91] So, we're not getting farther away from the Monsanto-driven reality of all this "wait-and-see" approach to the corn we're putting in both pet and human foods. We are embracing it at a rapid pace. And it's not just corn that is being raised GMO. From the Non-GMO Project, we retrieve the following list of crops affected (updated December of 2011):

- **Alfalfa** (first planting 2011)
- **Canola** (approx. 90% of U.S. crop)
- **Corn** (approx. 88% of U.S. crop in 2011)
- **Cotton** (approx. 90% of U.S. crop in 2011)
- **Papaya** (most of Hawaiian crop; approximately 988 acres)

- **Soy** (approx. 94% of U.S. crop in 2011)
- **Sugar Beets** (approx. 95% of U.S. crop in 2010)
- **Zucchini and Yellow Summer Squash** (approx. 25,000 acres)…
- **Beta vulgaris** (e.g., chard, table beets)
- **Brassica napa** (e.g., rutabaga, Siberian kale)
- **Brassica rapa** (e.g., bok choy, mizuna, Chinese cabbage, turnip, rapini, tatsoi)
- **Cucurbita** (acorn squash, delicata squash, patty pan)
- **Flax**
- **Rice**
- **Wheat**[92]

Using corn as an example, if a dog or cat food label lists corn in the ingredients, what are the chances that the corn was derived from the 15 percent of acreage devoted to non-GMO practice? With all the strong debate regarding the risks of GMO ingredients and our nation's green groups primarily focused on the health and wellness of humans above pets (which it should be), wouldn't a much larger focus be placed on using the unaffected corn crops for human food instead of pet food? And with so much focus on human health, is anybody really paying attention specifically to GMOs as they relates to the pet food industry?

We know for sure that the FDA, once again, doesn't seem to care. From the Non-GMO Project website, we read:

Unfortunately, even though polls consistently show that a significant majority of Americans want to know if the food they're purchasing contains GMOs, the powerful biotech lobby has succeeded in keeping this information from the public.[93]

And from the FDA website, we read that although they claim to regulate GMO crops and consider them "safe" (regardless of the conflicting information in this section of the chapter), they do *not* require any food labels—pet or human—to divulge this information.

Many consumers are interested in knowing whether the food they serve their families [or pets] is produced using genetic engineering. Food manufacturers may indicate through *voluntary* labeling whether foods have or have not been developed through genetic engineering, provided that such labeling is truthful and not misleading....

Food labeling is misleading if it fails to reveal "material" facts—information that is material in light of statements made or suggested on the label, or material with respect to consequences that may result from the use of the food.[94]

The following is a list of ingredients derived from GMO crops:

Amino Acids, Aspartame, Ascorbic Acid, Sodium Ascorbate, Vitamin C, Citric Acid, Sodium Citrate, Ethanol, Flavorings ("natural" and "artificial"), High-

Fructose Corn Syrup, Hydrolyzed Vegetable Protein, Lactic Acid, Maltodextrins, Molasses, Monosodium Glutamate [MSG], Sucrose, Textured Vegetable Protein (TVP), Xanthan Gum, Vitamins, Yeast Products.[95]

Several of these ingredients have been reported to cause adverse effects in pets, and it would take an entire chapter to break down which are harmful, and why. As the reader is most likely aware, this is a book written to provide evidence of poor practice in the industry, not to scientifically educate each reader with the exhaustive approach of a medical or scientific textbook. Therefore, we will address just a few:

Ethanol:

Ethanol poisoning (toxicosis) [within pets] occurs from exposure to the chemical ethanol, either orally or through the skin, and results most commonly in a depression of the central nervous system—expressed in the animal as drowsiness, lack of coordination or unconsciousness. Other effects may include damage to body cells, and symptoms such as incontinence, slowed heart rate, and even heart attack.[96]

High-Fructose Corn Syrup, Sucrose, and Molasses:

Any HFCS, sucrose, or molasses found in the original GMO crop is only an additive to what many pet food manufacturers are already placing in their pet foods during the cooking process. The sugary taste of HFCS certainly entices the animal to eat quickly, giving pet owners a reason to believe the food is being enjoyed—and some sources credit this ingredient as an assistant toward better end-product "texture"[97]—but HFCS, as well as sucrose (and molasses in excess), is just as bad for pets as it is for humans.

> Continuous intake can promote hypoglycemia, obesity, nervousness, cataracts, tooth decay, arthritis and allergies. Pets also get addicted to foods that contain sugars, so it can be a tough piece of work to make them eat something healthier.[98]

It is also worthy to note that sorbitol "is the alcohol of sucrose. Intestinal absorption is poor for sorbitol and excessive amounts can result in diarrhea."[99]

Hydrolyzed Vegetable Protein, Textured Vegetable Protein (TVP), and Monosodium Glutamate (MSG):

MSG is another ingredient that is both directly added to the GMO crops as well as to the pet foods during the commercial pet food manufacturing process. It is a flavor enhancer and an addictive substance (which can keep your pet addicted to these bad foods).[100]

> The MSG in pet foods [is] created chemically by either *hydrolyzing vegetable protein* [or *Textured Vegetable Protein*] (almost always from soy) or fermenting glucose

from starches.... MSG tricks the tongue receptors into thinking food is higher in protein than it actually is. It actually excites brain cells into making them over-react to substances. In the over-reactive state, the dog or cat consuming it believes the food tastes better. This allows pet food companies to use lower quality proteins and other low quality ingredients and fillers....

Neither the U. S. Food and Drug Administration (USDA) nor the American Association of Feed Control Officers (AAFCO) require MSG be listed on the ingredient labels of pet foods. Instead it may appear as hydrolyzed protein, natural flavoring, natural liver flavoring, yeast extract, hydrolyzed corn gluten or liver digest.

MSG can:
- Stimulate or damage the nervous system
- Create taurine deficiencies
- Damage brain cells
- Affect the thyroid
- Cause obesity[101]

Some of these ingredients will come up again later in this book. This short list is only included to educate the reader that if a pet food contains ingredients originating from GMO crops (which do *not* have to be labeled as such, according to the FDA), there is an entire other list of additives synthetically meshed with the original crops, which, secondary to the GMO crops themselves, do not have to be labeled. Put simply, the crops, themselves, do not have to be shown on any label as

GMO, and with every GMO product comes an entire list of inherited ingredients from the original crop—ingredients that will never show on the label.

Because of the lack of regulation regarding the labeling of ingredients as genetically modified, it would be impossible to know whether the pet food you are purchasing is free of all these risks, unless the food is verified as non-GMO. More pet food manufacturers are becoming GMO-free, so keep an eye out for those foods specifically labeled as such. Also keep in mind that a GMO-free-labeled food may mean that it contains non-GMO crops and even tests as non-GMO, but it can still contain meat from food animals that were fed GMO crops their entire life. Although this may be slightly healthier, it can and will still transfer some harmful additives to your pet. So, how do you know if the food you are choosing is completely GMO-free? The food will specifically state "USDA Organic" on the packaging. This, at the time of this writing, is the healthiest and most certified approach to non-GMO foods for both you and your pet. Unfortunately, this certification is not yet on many pet food labels, but as pet owners become more demanding about their companions' health, more health-conscious companies are trying to the meet the demand. So, it's likely that we will see an increase in this notation on future pet food labels. (For additional information on the subject of non-GMO pet foods, and for a list of pet foods the Non-GMO Project states are verified as GMO-free, visit: "Verified Products: Pet Products," *Non-GMO Project*, last accessed June 11, 2015, http://www.nongmoproject.org/find-non-gmo/search-participating-products/?catID=51280730.)

The results of GMO ingredients in your pet's food bowl are hotly debated within the scientific community since the practice is still so new. However, one needs only to search the equivalent of "GMO pet food" in any online database to flood the computer monitor with hundreds of articles pointing to the permanent and generational terrors of GMO influence.

And, as it begs to be said, all of this hullabaloo about which grain is better than others within a pet's food seems less important than it should be, considering that dogs and cats generally don't need grains, anyway.

No Grains?

Because there has been so much talk in our society regarding the controversy in human dietary needs for carbohydrates, it shouldn't come as a shock that facts about carbohydrates are even more obscure to the general public in regard to pet foods. It goes back to the same standard rule that people pay a lot more attention to human foods than to pet foods. Dogs and cats, when fed properly, will have a healthy supply of water, protein, and some fats well before they are given carbohydrates. It should not be assumed that natural (non-GMO) grains or corn are inherently *bad* for your pet, but the public is largely unaware that these ingredients are not at all among the most primary nutritional needs. Many veterinarians acknowledge that a certain amount of grains and carbohydrates are beneficial to a cat or dog, but are never at the top of the list.

But don't take our word for it. Let's take a look at some

highly reputable pet-wellness and veterinary sources regarding the nutritional need for grains and carbohydrates in canine and feline diets. In *Canine and Feline Nutrition: A Resource for Companion Animal Professionals*, Linda Case—a canine nutritionist, dog trainer, and science writer who earned her BS in animal science at Cornell University and her MS in canine/feline nutrition at the University of Illinois—acknowledges that the question of grains in pet foods is almost irrelevant in today's world. "The fact that dogs and cats do not require carbohydrates is immaterial," she says, "because the nutrient content of most commercial foods include [carbohydrates]."[102] In other words, you're likely going to get a food with grains at or near the top of the ingredients list regardless of what brand of food you buy your pet, *if* you buy your pet a commercial food. So, starting with a commercial brand is unwise if you're looking to avoid unnecessary filler material and really hone in on your animal's true nutritional needs. Mark Morris Sr. (founder of the celebrated and now-controversial Science Diet) even acknowledges this to be true when he says, "Some question exists regarding the need of dogs and cats for dietary carbohydrate. From a practical sense, the answer to this question is of little importance because there are carbohydrates in most food ingredients used in commercially prepared dog foods."[103]

And who are we to argue with or make a big deal about a matter of such "little importance"?

That is, unless, we want to provide our pets with the nutrients their species need, in which case, it suddenly becomes highly important—and Morris' comment seems ironically irrational. The truth is, if you are feeding your pet a commercial food, he or she is getting far more grains than needed, and in many cases, far more than he or she will ever be able to digest, which only leads to looser, smellier stools consisting of many substances the animal's digestive tracts have rejected. This issue is also far worse with dry foods than with wet, canned foods. Natural Pet Productions states, "The natural, ancestral diet of dogs and cats included minimal amounts of grain, yet even the 'healthiest' dry foods are half grain."[104]

How many carbohydrates does your companion really need? *The Waltham Book of Companion Animal Nutrition* says, "There is no known minimum dietary requirement for carbohydrate."[105]

Another discouraging fact: Protein content (the listed percentage of protein within a food as it relates to the nutrition facts on a label) can be hidden in vegetable and plant proteins instead of meat sources. For example, there are proteins in your hair. If a pet food company added hair to the mix, they could claim the proteins from the hair as adding to the percentage of available proteins in the food, but that does *not* mean that it's a healthy source of protein *or* that the protein is even digestible. From a purely scientific standpoint, the verdict on the myth of vegetable and plant proteins is out. According to T. J. Dunn, DVM of Pet MD:

> It is common knowledge and generally agreed upon by experts that dogs (and cats) are meat eaters and have evolved through the ages primarily as meat eaters. Although now "domesticated," our pets have not

evolved rumens along their digestive tracts in order to ferment cellulose and other plant material, nor have their pancreases evolved a way to secrete cellulase to split the cellulose into glucose molecules, nor have dogs and cats become efficient at digesting and assimilating and utilizing plant material as a source of high quality protein. Herbivores do those sorts of things. That's how nature is set up at this time.[106]

But for those readers who know little about "rumens along digestive tracts," "fermenting cellulose," "evolved pancreases," or "cellulase secretions," and have no interest in or time to self-educate on the complicated science behind canine and feline digestive history, perhaps a simpler explanation is needed. From Only Natural Pet, we read:

The truth is that high *plant* protein diets are hard on your pet's organs; high animal protein diets aren't only healthy for your aging pets, but essential. Poor quality, mass produced pet foods are packed with protein from soy and corn. Unfortunately, your dog and cat are unable to properly digest and assimilate these sources of protein. It lets the food manufacturer boost the protein content of the food without actually offering your pet any substantial protein they can use. High plant protein diets can put added strain on your pets because their bodies aren't designed to process those ingredients. As they try to assimilate protein from these sources, their organs need to start working overtime.… When choosing a healthy, high protein diet for your pet, avoid any bags that feature corn or soy as a prominent ingredient (or better yet, avoid them all together). You want named meat meals (like chicken meal or lamb meal) or quality meat as the primary protein source. This is a sureproof way to make sure your pets are eating the diet nature intended.[107]

If your pet is currently sick, it *may* have less to do with the fact that you're serving him a grains-based diet, and more to do with the fact that the grains-based diet probably lacks the actual nutrition the pet needs in the first place. It would be similar to wondering why a human is sick when all he has eaten is straight vegetarian pasta for the last several years. Maybe he has taken great pains to ensure that the grains he has put into his body have come from non-GMO, natural, and nutrient-packed sources. It wouldn't matter. For a human, it's not that the source of the carbohydrate has been compromised, it's the fact that the person has lived *without* all other essential nutrients derived from fruits, vegetables, and proteins for years. Humans and pet companions have extremely different dietary needs, but one trait we share is that we need more than the excess of one source ingredient to sustain great health. If the food you are giving Fido and Fluffy has a grain listed as the first ingredient, and some of the protein content is hidden within even more grains, the other nutrients will never be as high as they need to be for a cat or dog.

In conclusion: We should remember that grains, although typically considered a "filler" ingredient by most professionals in the field of canine and feline health, are not always directly the source of most pet health problems, assuming the grains are naturally produced and clean (but see the following pages). Lack of proper proteins and other essential nutrients is a factor, but even this pales in comparison to the poor meat sources appearing in pet foods across the globe. If your pet is getting less-than-ideal amounts of meat-sourced protein in his or her diet, and the meat-sourced protein he or she *is* getting is of poor quality (such as those addressed in the previous chapter), *and* the food contains foreign materials that no mammal should be ingesting (also addressed in previous chapter), then grain content is not the first thing that should be adjusted. Correcting the proteins is a first and foremost focus. Dr. Ken Tudor of Pet MD said it well:

> Pet foods contain many low quality products. There are only *quantity*, and not *quality* standards for pet food. That is why carcasses in any stage of decomposition are acceptable for pet foods. Animals in any stage of dying (down, disabled, and dying for whatever reason) are acceptable. Tissue levels of any drug, including euthanasia solution, are acceptable for pet food. There are even acceptable limits for sawdust, nut shells, beaks, claws, scales, bones, rodent contamination, and plastic bag particles for pet food. So why quickly blame grain…for digestive problems?[108]

Harm in Excess

Before we leave this thread on grains, one thing must be clear: Although grains are seen by many as harmless to cats and dogs in moderation, a lot of research is available to one who fairly wants to compare the harm of occasional grains versus constant grains. In excess, grain sources in pet foods have been linked to many growing health concerns. Recall that we spoke of a sharp increase in cancer in domestic pets within recent decades. Could it be that grains hold a significant responsibility in the development of cancer?

Grains are packed with carbohydrates. Once ingested, carbohydrates convert to sugar. Sugar feeds cancer cells. Creating a cancer-feeding environment within a pet certainly increases the chances of cancer growth.[109]

And sadly, it doesn't stop there. From The Whole Dog, we read:

> Grains and or grain based foods are, also, the main cause of yeast infections, such as Candida Albicans in our pets. Symptoms of yeast over-growth or infections include:
> —habitual scratching, usually the ears, sides of the torso and underbelly
> —chronic ear infections
> —incessant licking of the genitals or the paws or both
> —lick granulomas
> —rashes, most often on the underbelly
> —hair loss

—blackening and rough skin patches

—Allergies (so called)

—and when the yeast begins to move into the head; loss of hearing; loss of eyesight; loss of intelligence, memory and comprehension.[110]

Dr. Elizabeth Hodgkins, DVM, also states: "A highly processed, grain-based diet fed to an animal designed to thrive on a meat-based, fresh food diet is very likely to produce symptoms of ill health over time. Diets to address disease most frequently deal with the symptoms that are the result of a lifetime of inappropriate food, not the true cause of their symptoms."[111]

This all traces back to the excess of anything a body doesn't need within that body's daily diet. When an animal is given poor (commercial) foods, that animal is going to experience poor health conditions. When the pet owner takes that animal to a veterinary care professional to assess his or her condition, the *symptoms* are frequently treated before the *cause* of the symptoms. The pet owner then takes the animal home, and continues to feed the pet food that, to the trained/educated eye, appears to be manufactured specifically for making animals sick with terrible proteins and useless, nutrient-devoid "filler" scraps.

What's worse, when considering excess, is the *quality* of the grains included in pet foods. After the harvest of a grain source, that source must be stored, and sometimes for very lengthy periods, before it is used. During the storage process, many contaminants play a factor in the overall quality of the original harvest, including "hulls, chaff, straw, dust, dirt, and sand swept from the mill floor at the end of each week,"[112] as well as "insects, mites, [and] mold."[113] The stored grains that have reached beyond the grain contaminant levels deemed fit for human consumption are easily accepted into the pet food industry for consumption by our lesser species.

A single grain mite, a close cousin to the dust mite (responsible for numerous allergy problems in humans), can lay up to eight hundred eggs in just over a week.[114] It's little wonder that the longer the grains remain in storage, the more infested they can become with disease- and allergy-causing mites. One common, but miserable, allergy-related disease in canines is atopic dermatitis. Symptoms include:

- skin lesions (caused by chronic scratching)
- scaly skin
- skin infections
- red, inflamed skin
- red or brown staining on skin (or black near the genitals)
- hair loss
- signs of excessive itching, scratching, rubbing, or licking anywhere, but especially near face, paws, belly, groin, and underarms

Many, including veterinary professionals, have claimed that household dust mites are the central cause of this condition, but recent studies show otherwise. In a scientific study conducted by Wright State University called "Serum Immunoglobulin E against Storage Mite Allergens in Dogs with

Atopic Dermatitis," we read that "storage mite sensitivity in dogs may be as important, if not more important, than dust mite sensitivity."[115]

This report indicates that storage mites and their contribution to one of the most common conditions in canines are merely one of many conceivable consequences originating from the excess of poor-quality grains. Additionally, this study is only on *one* of the insects found in stored grains. A more complete list would mention the following, all of which are in the "common" category (an exhaustive list would include the "uncommon" mites found in grains also, but that list is so long it cannot be included here):

- Granary weevil (*Sitophilus granarius*)
- Rice weevil (*Sitophilus oryzae*)
- Maize weevil (*Sitophilus zeamais*)
- Bean weevil (*Acanthoscelides obtectus*)
- Pea weevil (*Bruchus pisorum*)
- Southern cowpea weevil (*Callosobruchus chinensis*)
- Larger grain borer (*Prostephanus truncatus*)
- Lesser grain borer (*Rhyzopertha dominica*)
- Rust-red flour beetle (*Tribolium castaneum*)
- Confused flour beetle (*Tribolium confusum*)
- Large flour beetle (*Tribolium destructor*)
- Sawtoothed grain beetle (*Oryzaephilus surinamensis*)
- Merchant grain beetle (*Oryzaephilus mercator*)
- Flat grain beetle (*Cryptolestes spp.*)
- Rusty grain beetle (*Cryptolestes ferrugineus*)
- Flour mill beetle (*Cryptolestes turcicus*)

- Khapra beetle (*Trogoderma granarium*)
- Indian meal moth (*Plodia interpunctella*)
- Tropical warehouse moth (*Ephestia cautella*)
- Angoumois grain moth (*Sitotroga cerealella*)
- Cadelle (*Tenebroides mauritanicus*)
- Mould mite (*Tyrophagus putrescentiae*)
- Flour mite (*Acarus siro*)
- Straw-itch mite (*Pymotes tritici*)

Now consider that even in addition to all these listed insects and mites is their droppings. Yes, their "poop." Yet, as gross is that sounds, it is still the tip of the iceberg.

As these pests swarm the stored grains for hours, days, weeks, and months on end, they become content little carriers of an invisible poison: mold. Although mold can and often does travel by air, in a stored grain bin where air is not as much of a factor, the contamination of the grain by mold depends widely upon carrier bugs. And we're not talking about a big, fuzzy, green splotch like what you would see on a bread loaf that you've kept for too long in your bread box. These spores are invisible to the naked eye.

As the mold seeps into all the grain, it produces myco-toxins. We can read more about mycotoxins in a study of the same name published by the US National Library of Medicine within the National Institutes of Health. From the abstract of that review, we read:

Mycotoxins are secondary metabolites produced by microfungi that are capable of *causing disease and death* in humans and other *animals*. Because of their pharmacological activity, some mycotoxins or myco-toxin derivatives have found use as antibiotics, growth promotants, and other kinds of drugs; still others have been implicated as chemical warfare agents. This review focuses on *the most important ones associated with human and veterinary diseases,* including afla-toxin, citrinin, ergot akaloids, fumonisins, ochratoxin A, patulin, trichothecenes, and zearalenone.[116]

The risks each of these mycotoxins represents to our pet companions are devastating. Conditions caused by a poison-ing often do lead to death, and those deaths are frequently misunderstood by the veterinary circles as "mysterious disease" or "rare disease" and misdiagnosed as other illnesses. Symp-toms of exposure can include vomiting, high fevers, blood in the stool, diarrhea, jaundice, and off-colored or dark urine. If all of these symptoms are present, a "mysterious disease" might be diagnosed. But how often does a veterinary care pro-fessional take a vomiting dog seriously? Because this kind of illness is usually the last thing a veterinary professional would ever suspect, the pet goes home to eat more poison.

But that hardly ever happens, right? Mycotoxin-related poi-sonings must be rare, or else pets would be dying all over the place because of this...right?

Actually, it happens more often than you think. "Aflatoxin toxicosis"—a condition related directly to mycotoxin-contam-inated grains—has been the leading reason for past pet food recalls, and it's deadly. According to the Oregon Veterinary

Medical Association, "Aflatoxin toxicosis is an occasional reason for recalls of our pets' foods.... Aflatoxins can cause considerable damage to the cells that make up the liver. One of the aflatoxins that can be found in pet foods is called aflatoxin B1.... Signs that your pet might be suffering from aflatoxin toxicosis include: lethargy, weakness, loss of appetite, vomiting, bloody diarrhea or black-tarry stool, yellow mucous membranes and possibly seizures." The organization goes on to describe the treatment of this illness: "Treatment is strictly supportive and may include fluid therapy, hospitalization, anti-vomiting medication, stomach protectants, plasma transfusions, Vitamin K1 treatments, IV antibiotics and liver specific treatments, such as SAMe (a hepatoprotectants)." That is, of course, a costly medical treatment that could have been avoided by sparing our pets from eating grain-based foods every day. Also note, "There is no specific antidote for aflatoxin toxicosis."[117] In this article alone, we have read of a terrible, costly, miserable condition of which there is no known cure—all originating from a grains harvest that was contaminated during storage.

So, are "grains" an enemy of Fido and Fluffy? Not necessarily. It's the quality and excess of the grains that raise a risk.

Would it surprise you with all the research we have presented thus far about the types of poor ingredients the pet food industry is willing to utilize to save themselves a buck, that the most infested crops—those deemed unfit for human consumption—then become the cheapest grain stocks, and therefore, the best choice for greedy pet food manufacturers?

Grain is not the immediate enemy. Lack of proper nutrition all around, with the addition of harmful ingredients, is the enemy.

We have looked at some of the harmful ingredients that appear in commercial pet foods as a result of crazy meat handling at rendering plants, as well as how grains can affect our companions. The following section will take a closer look at some of the specific ingredients listed on the food labels, how those ingredients play a role in our pets' health, and what we should be looking for when considering our pets' individual needs.

Red-Flag Ingredients[118]

Many ingredients in pet foods that cause health concerns are not even placed in the foods for nutritional purposes to begin with, including, but not limited to, preservatives, dyes, flavorings, and sweeteners, as well as additives that help with consistency and moisture rating.

The following is a list of these ingredients. (Please note that the following material is not exhaustive. We have included this information to raise awareness of only a small list of dangers that are frequently overlooked. If a pet owner has a pet with special needs, current illnesses, questions regarding a specific ingredient not listed below, or any follow-up needs regarding further information on food labels, these authors strongly suggest that the reader obtain additional research materials. One book that we would highly suggest is the large and well-organized book, *Dr. Pitcairn's Complete Guide to Natural*

Health for Dogs and Cats. It was written by a DVM, PhD, and covers almost every imaginable ailment, exhaustive information on label-reading, specialized diets, and routine medical treatment from a holistic perspective—and it even includes a section on how to say goodbye to a beloved animal whose health is failing or who has recently passed.)

Preservatives

In normal food practice, preservatives are good when they are natural. Without preservatives, food can become rancid and poisonous. However, unnatural preservatives can cause, and *have* caused, unbelievable health hazards. Here are a few preservatives commonly used in pet foods today:

Butylated hydroxyanisole (BHA): Used in pet foods to preserve fats, oils, and flavorings.
- Known to cause tumors in animals
- Dramatically affects the reproductive system in rats
- Decreased growth in rats
- Increased mortality rates in rats
- Potential human carcinogen
- Listed as known carcinogen in the state of California
- Listed as GRAS by the FDA

Butylated Hydroxytoluene (BHT): Cousin to BHA, used in pet foods to preserve fats, oils, and flavorings.
- Poorly tested
- Shown to cause cancer in animals

- Linked to liver damage and liver tumors
- Linked to lung damage and lung tumors
- Some association with metabolic stress
- Some association with serum cholesterol increase
- Has caused developmental issues in rat testing associated with fetal abnormalities and thyroid abnormalities
- Has caused developmental issues in rat testing associated with motor skills and coordination
- Listed as GRAS by the FDA

Ethoxyquin: Originally Monsanto-developed as a rubber stabilizer and pesticide/herbicide used to preserve post-harvest fruits, as well as a color preservative. Used now in pet foods to assist with oxidation and prevent development of organic peroxides, it is largely considered one of the most dangerous preservatives in pet foods. It is also sometimes one of the most well-hidden ingredients, as it can be added to the meat/meal by-products prior to pet food manufacturing, and, therefore, would not always be listed on the pet food label.

- Widely linked to cancer in the liver, stomach, skin, and spleen
- Has caused liver tumors in mice
- Linked to liver-related illnesses
- Linked to thyroid-related illnesses
- Linked to kidney damage and kidney-related illness
- Linked to reproductive abnormalities
- Linked to immune-deficiency syndrome
- Linked to blindness

- Linked to leukemia
- Considered by many in science to be carcinogenic
- Not an approved preservative for pet food in Australia
- Not an approved preservative in the European Union
- Has never once been proven safe for the lifespan of a pet
- Currently under investigation regarding complications to blood and liver, yet still used as a preservative in US pet foods today

Propyl Gallate: Used as a fat stabilizer, propyl gallate can often be "snuck" into products via Vitamin C.

- Suspected of causing liver damage and liver diseases
- Linked to cancer
- Mimics estrogen, and therefore adversely effects the reproductive system, developing fetuses, and sperm count in males
- Can cause digestive upset
- Can cause stomach irritation
- Listed as GRAS by the FDA

Propylene glycol: Used in pet foods to stabilize moisture, inhibit bacterial growth, maintain texture, and as a sweetener, it is largely considered one of the most dangerous preservatives in pet foods. It also happens to be a well-known ingredient in antifreeze.

- Known to cause illness in canines
- Can inhibit the growth of an animal's "good" bacteria (because of its effects on the inhibition of bacterial growth)

- Can cause blockage or cancerous lesions in the intestines (because of its use in moisture control)
- Considered to cause the most overlooked issues in canine health, including itching, dryness of skin, dehydration, hair loss, anemia, and irregularities in the mouth (teeth, gums)
- Listed as GRAS by the FDA

Tertiary Butylhydroquinone (TBHQ): Used as a fat preservative in pet foods, as well as an ingredient in explosives, varnishes, resins, and lacquers.
- Contains petroleum-derived butane
- Linked to pre-cancerous stomach tumors in labs
- Can cause damage to DNA
- Considered safe by the FDA in certain food uses (pet food included)

Dyes

Dyes have no nutritional value. Their sole purpose is to appeal to the eye and convince consumers that the colorful products they are buying are fresh and pretty. In pet foods, dyes can also be deceptive in that they insinuate ingredients that aren't always present, or when they are present, are negligible in their nutritional contribution. Take kibble, for instance. How many times have you seen bags of chow with pictures on the front that show orange, red, yellow, green, tan, and dark brown kibbles? The bites are often shaped differently as well to look like carrots, tomatoes, apples, celery stalks, miniature steaks, and miniature dog bones, suggesting to the buyer a healthy balance of fruits and vegetables as well as protein—when, in reality, the entire mix of chow comes from one cooked batch and is simply dyed to suggest variety.

Like preservatives, some dyes have been historically linked to health hazards for animal feed as well as humans. Here is a short list of a few dyes that commonly appear in pet foods:

Red No. 3 (also known as erythrosine):
- Recognized by the FDA in 1990 to be a thyroid carcinogen in animals
- Currently banned for use in human cosmetics and topical drugs, but not in pet foods

Red No. 40:
- Most widely-used food dye
- A possible carcinogen
- Linked to cancer
- May accelerate immune system tumors in mice
- Widely associated with cancer-causing contaminants, as well as controversy surrounding ADHD and hyperactivity in human children

Yellow No. 5 (also known as tartrazine or E102):
- Second most widely-used food dye
- Derived from coal tar
- Not fully tested
- Possible carcinogen
- Linked to cancer

- Linked to thyroid tumors
- Linked to severe hypersensitivity
- Linked to neurochemical effects, including hyperactivity, insomnia, and aggression
- Linked to asthma
- Linked to lymphomas
- Linked to chromosomal damage
- A salicylate, which can become fatal to felines with extended use
- Strongly associated with allergic reactions
- Banned in some European countries
- Can only be used with a warning label in some European countries
- Associated with controversy surrounding ADHD and hyperactivity in human children

Yellow No. 6:
- Third most widely-used food dye
- Derived from petroleum
- Possible carcinogen
- Linked to cancer
- Linked to severe hypersensitivity
- Linked to asthma
- Linked to chromosomal damage
- Linked to skin issues
- Has caused tumors in the adrenal gland and kidney in animal testing
- Associated with allergic reactions
- Banned in several European countries

- Currently being eliminated from use in the UK
- Associated with controversy surrounding ADHD in human children

Blue No. 2:
- Possible carcinogen
- Links to brain tumors (chiefly brain gliomas), as well as abnormal brain cell development, in male mice and rats
- Studies have shown that canines have an increased sensitivity to deadly viruses
- Can contain cancer-causing contaminants

Flavorings

Very often, food labels simply refer to this as "artificial flavorings" or generically "flavoring." This could mean so many things that we could spend an entire chapter talking about it. To be brief, many times the flavorings within pet foods are cooked-down broths or tallow substances from rendering plant leftovers. Since we have already looked at those practices at length, we will not discuss it again here. However, it begs to be stated that if you are wary of the protein by-products you read about already, the same caution should apply when seeing generic flavoring listed on a pet food label. Flavorings can also be carcinogenic, and the regulations applied to them are even looser than with many other substances. Most often, the label will state the following terms: some variant of pyrophosphates, animal digest, digest, glandular meal, flavor, flavorings, and artificial flavoring.

Sweeteners

Obviously, sweeteners are not included in your pet's food for nutritional value. Sweeteners entice the senses of taste and smell. However, just like with humans, sweeteners can cause numerous health problems when used in excess. And remember that even though one feeding of a food with high levels of sweeteners likely wouldn't do any harm, giving sugary substances to a human or animal several times a day for years is naturally an excess. A constant supply of sweeteners to your pet can promote cancer growth, hyperactivity, and allergies, as well as cause hypoglycemia, diabetes, obesity, cataracts, and arthritis. All of this is in addition to how the sugars will eat away at your pet's teeth. Considering the addictive properties of sweeteners, a pet might also have a hard time transferring out of a sweeter diet and into a healthier one. Sweeteners can appear on the label in the following terms: sucrose, fructose, corn syrup, sugar, sorbitol, cane molasses, ammoniated glycyrrhizin, Dl-alpha tocopheryl acetate, and artificial sweeteners.

Conclusion

With all these terrible ingredients, and with so much pressure to make the right decision for your pet, you may feel tempted to call a professoinal for answers. Whereas some vets will recommend a certain brand of pet food, many will not, and there's a good reason for that.

In the next chapter we will visit the reason recommendations are not easy to come by, the different categories of pet diets, and how to better understand pet food labels.

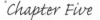

Chapter Five

Dietary Options
and Reading Labels

An ounce of prevention is worth a pound of cure.
—BENJAMIN FRANKLIN[119]

Diseases and health conditions are rampant in animal health care these days, and it doesn't seem to be getting any better across the board. Many veterinarians treat the symptoms of an illness or condition, but they don't always help the pet owner *prevent* the maladies—and prevention often starts with food. It is comparable to human medicine. For example, many obese men and women are placed on insulin for a diabetic condition caused by their obesity instead of being placed on a strict diet and exercise program to reduce their body mass and therefore decrease the need for insulin pills. Preventing a disease, illness, or condition through proper health is worth far more than curing or treating those issues later on.

Probably the most frequently asked question in veterinary medicine, as these authors have seen in their research as well as during conversations with DVMs, is, "What food should I buy for my pet?" Unfortunately, the issue is not that simple. First, you have to determine what your lifestyle can support in relation to the varying diets for pets; holistic veterinarians will likely suggest a home-prepared diet or raw diet, which differs enormously from any commercial diet. However, this can present complications for the pet owner. For example, someone with a full-time job, kids, and three large dogs may not be able to afford the time or money to prepare home-cooked dog meals in the kitchen. The elderly lady with a cat may have plenty of time and money to prepare her feline's meal, but she may not have the mobility it takes to do so. In these cases, owner-prepared meals might be ruled out. If either of these people has a strong conviction against a raw diet because of the associated salmonella risks, the natural option might be a more commercial diet. Barring the veterinarians who suggest a specific brand off the shelves of their own office stores as a result of their involvement in an incentives program, many vets (especially holistic) wouldn't recommend a commercial brand, even if better ones are available.

Why Commercial Food Brand Recommendations May Fail

One of these authors (Donna Howell, in this case) worked for an electronics specialty shop as one of her very first jobs. As she was being trained for a position on the sales floor, she was directed to a chart covering consumer reviews and customer feedback regarding the performance of well-known manufacturers of VCRs and televisions. The chart not only showed the current trends and leading manufacturers, but it also tracked their performance over the course of the company's history. One of the most recognized brands in the US, celebrated for its living-room entertainment endeavors, had erratic reviews, spiking and dipping over and over again for the past several decades. The chart for one year would indicate that nearly everyone who had bought the product loved it and only had wonderful things to say about its performance. The next year revealed a deep decline in the satisfaction surveys and a drop in the quality of the product. Then, there would be another rise. Although one particular brand demonstrated this pattern in the extreme, almost all major brands reported up-and-down waves in their products' consumer review history. This was confusing, so Donna asked for further clarification. The answer was enlightening.

As certain product manufacturers maintain only the highest quality, Donna's supervisor explained, they receive only the highest consumer reviews, because their products legitimately outperform the competitors. That brand becomes trusted by customers all over the world as the leading industry expert. That much was easy to follow. However, as these electronics companies gain clientele and become wealthier and wealthier as the industry's pros, they relax, knowing that anyone walking into a department store to pick up something for their living room will pay more for the trusted brands. They have "arrived." Then, their quality takes an extreme dip, resulting in less-than-ideal consumer reviews. Donna's trainer listed two potential reasons for this pattern:

1) The manufacturers *intentionally* drop their standards by cutting corners and using cheaper parts, cheating the public out of a worthy product while they float on a trusted name and make extemporaneous income on the machines they know in advance won't perform as promised. They take the risk, because their brand name is so trusted that they can skate for a good decade or so on cheap quality. When consumer reviews begin to taint their name, sales begin to drop, and the public starts turning to different brand names, these companies extract funds from the bank accounts that had grown during the sneaky era of cheating the public and launch new ad campaigns with new promises. These new promises are kept initially, earning back the public's trust. It doesn't need to be said that the minute they feel they are at the forefront of the industry, the cheating commences again. As it does, they continue to charge the highest prices for their products and advertise that it is the best on the market. Fancy marketing campaigns are nothing to them by this point, so deceiving the public is easy.

2) The manufacturers *unintentionally* drop their standards as a result of a change in ownership, financial difficulties, or a loss of ability to maintain cutting-edge approach to electronics that previously positioned them at the forefront of technology. Eventually they become the underachievers. Without the healthy bank accounts of the cheaters prior, they eventually become trusted in the industry for producing the "cheapest" products rather than the ones with the highest quality. Although many of the brands that fit into this category are still around, they are known for products that cost much less

initially and malfunction much earlier. Nonetheless, since money is a huge factor for many US consumers, this is a lucrative market to maintain.

This illustration not only applies to electronics, but also to the pet food industry. Because the industry is constantly changing and the moral standards and health education of any specific brand may dip at any time, the quality of a product endorsed today may not be the same tomorrow, and we may or may not know about it if or when that happens. This illustration also helps us understand why the most expensive product is certainly not always the best, and often it can be of less performance value than the lower-cost product on the market.

Thus, it is difficult for the authors of this book and for veterinary professionals who sincerely hold an interest in your pet's quality of life to recommend a commercial food source when, at any given moment, the right advice today can be the wrong advice tomorrow. The only fail-proof method of providing the best for an animal whose owner cannot adopt the lifestyle of preparing meals or offering raw meals is to help the pet owner understand what is on the label, and what should or should not be placed in Fido's bowl.

Three Categories of Diet

In order to decide what kind of diet is best for your animal, let's look at the three categories of diet: home-prepared, raw, and store-bought.

Home-Prepared

This diet offers both obvious and immediate benefits to every dog or cat. The owner has complete control of every ingredient in the food, and can therefore ensure that all the pet's nutritional needs are met. This method is certainly not as easy as buying commercial food, but it may end up being much simpler and more cost effective in the end than treating the illnesses that are often triggered by poorly manufactured commercial food. Additionally, since healthy pet-food ingredients are much easier to find than healthy ready-made pet foods, there is the added convenience of bypassing the nerve-wracking hunt for the perfect food label.

Note that the first thing to consider when it comes to home-prepared meals for your pet is that simply scraping what is left over on your plate into his bowl is *not* recommended. Although the pasta with meat sauce you're eating is likely going to be a step up from pet food that is otherwise derived from diseased meats in a rendering plant and moldy grains from harvest storage, it would not be considered a nutritionally balanced canine or feline meal. Over time, table scraps may keep your pet alive, but they won't ensure that he will thrive.

Yes, but dogs and cats lived just fine on table scraps back in the day, right?

Perhaps, but "back in the day," we didn't eat fattening foods riddled with artificials, synthetics, and sugars. Today, unless you live on a completely organic diet, the foods fit for human consumption aren't what they used to be. And if you *are* living on a completely organic diet, your pet still will not get the required amount of protein if you're giving him the last dollop of mashed potatoes, a few kernels of buttered corn, and one or two bites of chicken from your plate. Your pet will still be getting food that doesn't offer the nutrition, vitamins, supplements, etc., that he needs. For this reason, *some* veterinary professionals recommend avoiding home-prepared meals, for fear that the pet will become malnourished.

Recipes for home-prepared meals are appearing increasingly often in animal wellness literature and online. This is great news, as it represents the increase in concern for pet health. *It can also be alarming, however, because some of the recipes are written by well-meaning pet owners who do not have the knowledge or education to construct a recipe with an animal's exact biological needs in mind.* A cut of chicken leg with broccoli from a crock pot is not going to work. It's important to keep this in mind when looking for recipes.

As stated before, this book is primarily written to raise awareness of some of the controversial practices in the pet food industry. As a result, we have not included scientifically formulated recipes for you to cook at home. However, we can share a few tips about what to expect concerning home-cooked meals, if that is the route to which you feel drawn.

1. Remember to always choose organically raised ingredients. Keep in mind that harmful chemicals tend to sneak into products you wouldn't typically expect to find them in. As an example: If you decide to use peanut butter as an occasional source of protein

or as a fun treat, remember that it, too, must be organic, because nonorganic peanut butters typically have a tremendous amount of harmful additives and preservatives. (Notice that standard peanut butter almost never goes bad.) However, you will find that organic peanut butter is different than the leading commercial brands in that it will separate, sometimes causing a little more of a mess, requiring more stirring, and will need to be stored in your refrigerator. Further, because it doesn't include preservatives, it will have a shorter shelf life.

2. Steer clear of any ingredient sources that include artificial dyes, preservatives, or flavors.

3. The less the ingredients are processed, the easier it will be for your pet to digest and absorb the nutrients.

4. When choosing a meat, decide whether you will serve it cooked or raw (see the following section regarding raw diets). Fish, pork, or rabbit meat, as well as other exotic choices, must be cooked to kill off the parasites that these meats carry.

5. If you don't wish to use meat as a source of protein, consider using dairy products such as cottage cheese and eggs. (See *Dr. Pitcairn's Complete Guide to Natural Health for Dogs and Cats* for more information.)

6. Although fruits and vegetables are not more important than protein, they can provide essential vitamins and minerals, and should therefore be thoughtfully considered when planning a home-prepared meal for your pet.

7. Many pets will likely eat what you give them without much added flavor, simply because, unlike humans, they don't expect eating to provide a pleasant life experience. Unless they have grown accustomed to a lot of flavor, cats and dogs approach mealtime with more of a survival instinct: They eat to live and curb hunger. However, if your pet prefers more flavoring, there are a few natural ways to increase the palate temptation. For example, you can mix broth, broth powders, butter, tomato sauce, or fresh garlic into your pet's food dish. However, it's important to use these sparingly; whenever your pet *will* eat the food without these flavor enhancers, he should.

8. Any home-prepared meal should include vitamins and supplements suited to your pet's needs, especially calcium. Assuming your pet does not have special requirements, lists of standard vitamins or supplements are not hard to find, but this list *must* be obtained from a reliable and professional source such as a holistic veterinarian. Keep in mind that healthy fats and oils are also a must.

9. Make large batches of food at a time and freeze the extras for added convenience.

10. Always remember that if your pet was previously used to eating bagged kibble or canned food from a store, home-prepared meals will look, smell, and taste unfamiliar. Be patient when offering new dishes, and introduce them slowly, over a period of time, so as not to completely disrupt your pet's digestive system.

Also expect that his body may react to these different foods. If your pet turns away from the new diet at first, try warming up the food to encourage the switch. Also note that it's not uncommon for a pet to love his new diet at first, and then stop showing interest a few days later. Certain reactions to a new diet (such as lethargy, a seeming lack of appetite, passing worms, and other symptoms of internal cleansing from the previous commercial foods) can be alarming. Although some of this is to be expected, if you suspect your pet's health is suffering in any way or he is in danger, take him to a veterinarian. Much information is available regarding this transitional period, but it is important to acknowledge that changing from commercial foods to a home-prepared diet may require persistence and dedication.

If you decide to switch from a commercial diet to a home-prepared diet, consulting a holistic veterinarian should be one of the first steps you take. Regardless of where you get your recipes, what books you're reading, and whose advice you're following, if a trip to the vet ever becomes a necessity, partner with a professional who shares your passion for a holistic dietary approach. Don't be afraid to call around before making the transition, and find out who in your area will agree to work with you in getting your pet over the bumps, if there are any. Once you have a veterinary professional dialed in to your plan, gather all the necessary ingredients to begin and maintain the plan for a while. This will help you avoid putting your pet through a transition and then jerking him back to kibble for a month when your busy lifestyle doesn't provide opportunities to stock up, and then back again when you're better prepared.

Raw

This dietary method is a pretty hot-button topic in the veterinary world. There is a long list of debated pros and cons regarding feeding your animal raw meat. However, to fully understand all options of the raw diet, the reader must understand that there are two main philosophies behind it: the "prey-model" raw and the "prepared" raw.

In the former, the "prey-model," the pet is given an unadulterated, flesh-and-bone cut that appears exactly like a limb from a prey animal that has been hunted and killed in the wild. This is by far the closest simulation of a natural, wildlife diet. In the latter, the "prepared," meats are collected by a pet food company or a dedicated pet owner, then they are ground, mixed with vitamins, supplements, and minerals, and placed in a dish. Both diets are discussed here.

The Upsides:

1. **Mimics what nature intended:** A raw-meat diet most closely mimics the food sources that an animal in the wild would find and devour. This is the most obvious benefit to the raw diet, in most professional opinions.
2. **Promotes a more ideal weight:** Assuming that the meat obtained by the pet owner is clean, hormone-free, preservative-free, antibiotic-free, and free of all other

poor-choice ingredients (additives, dyes, etc.), this diet will have your pet consuming far more proteins, far more healthier fats, and far less carbohydrates than in even the best kibbles, keeping many pets at a more ideal weight. (Note that many commercially prepared raw diets contain meats that are USDA-inspected and are therefore similar, if not the same, as meats fit for human consumption.[120])

3. **Makes preparation simpler:** Another benefit is some of the ease at which this method can be carried out: no cooking is needed, there are no food labels to decipher, there are no concerns about loose and smelly stools (as much more of the needed nutrients are absorbed), and so on.

4. **Provides specific health advantages:** The diet will provide a means to a healthier digestion, skin, and coat, as well as a smaller chance of allergy issues.

5. **Offers added benefits:** If the prey-model raw diet is followed, a natural, hard bone is a follow-up treat to every meal, which provides additional nutrients, as well as (in many veterinary opinions) added teeth-cleansing and gum stimulation.

6. **Enhances recovery from illness:** Studies have also shown that pets suffering from sickness who are moved from commercial diets to the raw diet show an overall improvement in health.

The Downsides:

1. **Meat sources aren't always easy to come by.**
Constantly having to find healthy choice meat cuts

so often can be difficult at times. And, though raw pet diets are available in pet stores, major department stores (such as Walmart) may not have these foods in stock. (Note, however, that there are many online raw food diet stores, so if you are open minded about Internet shopping, you can purchase food online—without ever having to leave home.)

2. **Ensuring a balanced, nutritious meal can be difficult.** Because the raw-food diet sounds as easy as picking up a few extra meat selections on your next grocery trip, many well-meaning pet owners simply give their pets raw meat, still on the bone, straight from the supermarket fridge. But it's important to realize that the food animals your pet would consume in the wild are *also* wild, not "raised." They have probably been feeding on wild plants that have more nutrients than the cheap barn feeds that farm-raised animals eat. Additionally, when eaten in the wild, the source animal's entire body (including the stomach, with contents likely including vitamin-rich fruits or vegetables) is available for consumption, instead of just that "leg" in the fridge at the store. So simply feeding your pet a flesh-on-bone selection from a supermarket does not include the balanced meal rich with vitamins and minerals that your pet needs, unless you diligently provide those needs by other means. And since there is no way to know what nutrients are derivable from a store meat source, because the food animal was raised in a domestic feed setting, there remains a large hole

in your ability to ensure that your pet gets proper nutrition. Even if you were somehow able to get a hold of the rest of the food animal's remains, such as the stomach, there would be no way of knowing that the animal had been eating the same rich nutrients as a wild animal. Overall, the prey-model raw diet can sometimes deliver less-than-ideal nutrition results to well-meaning pet owners.

3. **Appropriate meat sources can be expensive.** As a contrast to number two above, if you wish to mimic the natural raw diet with meats that contain the vitamins, minerals, supplements, and scientific formulas necessary for optimal health, raw diet companies exist to make this far more convenient. However, not only does that place you in the position of having to find an appropriate food all over again and sift through all the companies that claim— for various reasons—to be the best, some of these companies charge a heavy price for these raw foods.

4. **Handling raw meat can be risky for humans.** Regardless of how "clean" the meat is that you obtain, any handling of raw meat has risks. The countertop, cutting surfaces, utensils, and most definitely your *hands* are all compromised, the same as when you handle any raw meat you prepare for your family. But what may not immediately occur to you is all the other surfaces the raw meat might contaminate. In the case of a prey-model diet, many animals carry off their food—and God only knows what all it will

touch before it's consumed. In both the prey-model and prepared diets, the pet's mouth contains bacteria from the raw meat, so whatever he licks or nuzzles up to is potentially contaminated. If the food touches your pet's coat—not an unlikely scenario—he can spread the bacteria to every surface he contacts. This is, in many professional opinions, a serious E. coli and salmonella threat to the humans who occupy the same space. (One horror story online noted that a toddler within the home followed his family dog down a hallway and was found a few minutes later eating the raw flesh from a leg of lamb alongside his pet. Certainly, pet owners who are parents should always keep a watchful eye on their children, but this story also illustrates that smaller children could be at greater risk even under the supervision of diligent parents. A contaminated binky, bottle, teething ring, toy, or blanket could be a breeding ground for dangerous bacteria.) This brings us to the question of the E. coli and salmonella threat to the pet.

5. **Eating raw meat might be risky for pets.** The number-one argument that pings back and forth in the ongoing health benefits-and-risks debate of the raw diet is the threat to the animal who eats the raw meat. On one hand, many veterinarians take the stance that canines and felines were created (either by God or evolutionary means) to scavenge from raw meat sources, and, therefore, their stomachs are not as vulnerable to the risks of E. coli and salmonella

poisoning. In addition, these pro-raw veterinarians suggest that any commercial brand of dog or cat food likely has a certain quantity of E. coli and salmonella as well, so the pet owners are not doing themselves or their pets any favors by feeding kibble to avoid this. (There is much reason to believe that this is true, considering the finds we referenced in earlier portions of the book regarding the FDA's response to salmonella detected in pet food.) On the other hand, professional veterinary opinion as well as common sense points to the fact that no person or animal is 100 percent impervious to the risks of illnesses brought on by the consumption of raw meat. Therefore, the possibility of a pet becoming extremely ill as a result of eating a raw diet is always present, even if the chances are much lower than in humans.

6. **Raw meats might be infected.** An additional debate rages between veterinarians over the threat to the pet regarding eating meats infected by worms, parasites, and unidentified pathogens. On one hand, a pet that consumes infected raw meat could become very ill, the consequences of which could possibly lead to death. On the other hand, pro-raw veterinarians typically state that these risks are preventable. According to these claims, infected meats frozen or cooked at specific temperatures for certain lengths of time (depending on the original meat source) can lose their harmful properties. The statements on both

sides of this argument are typically highly scientific and demand a lot more space than we can provide here. But hopefully this is enough to help educate the readers of issues they should be ready to approach with caution and care for the safety of their pet.

7. **Bone fragments can cause problems.** Lastly, specific to the prey-model raw diet, there is a risk that chewing on a raw bone can lead to small bone chips and sharp fragments making their way through the digestive system. This could result in painful and hazardous internal lesions, as well as accumulation of bone mass, causing blockage along the digestive tract. In some extreme cases, surgical removal of this mass would be necessary.

Despite all the risks, many pro-raw veterinarian professionals who have been in practice for decades have claimed that pets on raw diets have never experienced any of the above issues while in their care. These authors wish to make each reader aware of what the ongoing statements are from one professional to another. By no means do we intend to propagate or dismiss any risks to your pet. If you are strongly considering a switch to the raw diet, as with the home-prepared diet, your first step should be to consult a veterinary professional who shares your interest in this endeavor, and who will agree to treat your pet should problems arise. (Also note what Dr. Jean Hofve has to say in the section: "Interview with a Holistic Veterinarian.")

Store-Bought

Much of this book has referred to "commercial" diets as negative. This is because so many consumers pay for pet food that deceives with fancy advertising and false claims, and which has been manufactured with almost no regulation. However, although they are rare and sometimes hard to find, some healthier pet foods (especially canned) *can* be bought in stores or boutiques. They frequently cost around the same as many of the commercial brands that make amazing claims and fall short of delivery, so before you assume that the healthier foods will be too expensive, consider:

1. Many terrible and nutritionally void foods considered by the uninformed public to be the "high-end" choices are actually *more expensive* than the healthier foods you can find in specialized stores or boutiques.

2. Because the healthiest of store-bought choices provide much more nutrition for your pet instead of indigestible fillers, your pet needs far less food at each feeding. This means that even *when* the healthier bag is more expensive, it really isn't more costly in the long run, because the food will stretch farther. And for pet owners who are currently feeding their pets an expensive—but nutritionally deficient—food (as is the case with many commercial brands that claim their food is the best when it's not), switching to a truly healthier brand actually saves quite a bit of money.

As with the home-prepared and raw diets described in the previous pages, if your pet has been living on a bad diet for a long time, switching from that bad food to a healthier one *may* require a bit of a transitional process at the beginning. However, the shift from a bad commercial diet to a much better, store-bought diet shouldn't be hard to overcome, and it's most likely that a veterinarian's intervention won't be needed (although it certainly never hurts to have a vet on your side, no matter what healthcare changes you are administering to your pet).

As an example: Recently, a friend of these authors decided to switch his dog from a terrible commercial diet to a healthier kibble choice, based upon information we shared with him. At first, his dog devoured the new food without restraint, loving it, and speeding to her tray with her tail wagging each time she heard the bag rustling from the feed closet. She couldn't seem to get enough, so, for the first three or four days, our friend gave the dog the same amount of food that she had been given before the switch.

By about day five, our friend started to notice extra food in the dish after feeding, and this slowly started to stack up. At one of the dog's feedings, our friend noticed that the food hadn't been touched since the last time he had placed food in her bowl earlier that day. Worried that his dog had suddenly decided she didn't like the new food after all, he spoke to Joe (one of the authors of this book). Joe suggested that his friend cut back on the amount of food he was serving. Because the new food was much richer in nutrient content, the dog was being filled more efficiently, and simply didn't need the same amount of food twice per day as she had been given before.

Our friend cut down the food portions just a little, but still, food was left in the dish. So, he decreased the portions several more times, and, after about a week or so, the portions had been cut in half.

The next time Joe received an update about his friend's dog, it was positive. Not only does she now run to her dish with extreme excitement at each meal, but her coat has a new sheen, she has a substantial increase in energy and playfulness, and her stools are far more manageable. In addition to this good news, the owner's spending *has not* increased significantly. In fact, he buys smaller bags of food and feeds his dog half as much as before—for about the same as it cost for the previous brand's larger bags. (Please note that the healthier dry foods are free of dangerous preservatives, and therefore, do not have as long a shelf life as lower-quality foods. Pet owners should consider how fast the pet will go through the food when choosing the size of the bag.)

So, how do you find a better choice?

Whether you are solely relying on a store-bought pet food or you only plan to resort to the store-bought method when the home-prepared or raw diet is not practical for a specific event or time period, reading a pet food label doesn't have to be an enigmatic and frustrating affair, assuming you are willing to put forth a little time and practice. A few quick truths about labeling will help you make better choices for your pet.

Excessive Confusing Terminology Often Equals a Poor Product

As stated repeatedly throughout this book, pet food companies can and will use very confusing lingo on their labels, often relating to terminology that is never clearly defined by regulations, and they claim fantastic benefits of their brand with creative marketing to lure in a pet owner's trust. If a commercial food label uses words that only a scientist can understand, it's likely to be hiding a lot of bad ingredients within all that complicated text. The more jargon there is on the label, the more the buyer is forced to make a decision based on the company's claims and how appealing the packaging is, as opposed to making an informed decision about how the pet food relates to his pet's individual needs. Here's a good piece of advice: If you can't clearly understand most of the ingredients (especially the first several) on the label, put it back on the shelf.

Avoid the Obvious Red Flags

Meat: Many labels have some form of by-product listed. Meat by-products are the parts of a food animal that are not meat, such as organs, hooves, cow udders, beaks, etc. Rendering plants use the entire animal (as discussed earlier), and protein sources derived from rendering plants are commonly used in pet foods. When reading a label, the meat must be clearly identifiable as an animal, such as chicken, beef, lamb, buffalo, etc. A label listing "meat and bone meal," "meat meal," or something equivalent does not identify the animal of the sourced meat. Additionally, these components may be much harder to digest and offer much less nutritional value. Even terms such as "chicken by-product" and "beef by-product" don't indicate the source; these by-products may have come from a chicken or cow, but the fact that they are by-products (not meat) mean that Fido may be getting more beaks and hooves than breasts and thighs. Because of the importance of protein in your pet's diet, the meat source(s) should be the first thing on the label.

Corn and grains: As a general rule, any label that lists corn as a first ingredient can be eliminated. Such a food contains entirely too many carbohydrates and grains, and the protein content is much lower than your pet needs. In the same way that you should not tolerate by-products in the meat category, you should also think twice about any brand listing a by-product of grains. These may appear generically as "wheat millrun," "dried grains," "corn gluten meal," "brewers dried grains," "wheat middlings," and "bran." Not only are these grain by-products often sourced from the floors of grain manufacturing facilities (containing who knows what), but they can also come from "cereal food fines," the rejects and particles of breakfast cereals collected as debris during manufacturing. And, according to the Dog Food Advisor, "Cereal fines are lower quality ingredients that have been excluded from use in the human food industry."[121]

Preservatives and Dyes: In the last chapter, we covered some of the most alarming chemical additives appearing in pet food labels all over the world. Many of the mysterious illnesses (as well as common illnesses occurring for mysterious reasons) and deaths among cats and dogs today have been linked to these ingredients. The longer the shelf life of a pet food, the more likely it is that the food contains harmful preservatives. The more colorful the pet food, the more likely it is that the food contains harmful dyes. Avoid any label including the preservatives or dyes listed in the previous chapter.

Label Examples

At the time of this writing, there are two specific dry dog foods available in stores that stand as great examples of a company that uses terrible ingredients and a company with much higher nutrient standards. *We will not reveal the true name brands of the foods*, but we will compare what they contain to give you a better understanding of why you should immediately dismiss one and why the other deserves your consideration.

First, let's take a look at what these brands immediately present to the public.

The first brand, which we will simply refer to in this comparison as "Yum Yum's Poison Chow," is available in grocery stores and department stores all over the place, sells by the trainloads, and unabashedly lists some of the worst ingredients these authors have ever seen. The front of the bag, *of course*, shows a happy adult dog standing alert, its tongue wagging deliciously, just above several impressive-sounding claims about the food, including the infamous "Complete and Balanced," and other sought-after eye-candy such as "Vitamins and Minerals" (as if a pet food *wouldn't* otherwise contain vitamins and minerals).

The second, which we will call "Good Guy's Recipe Kibble," is, in this area, only available in veterinary clinics or specialized pet stores and pet boutiques, many of which cater to a more holistic-minded pet owner clientele. The front of the bag, surprisingly, is incredibly modest, showing no happy dog photos, men in lab coats, nor catchy sales slogans. The words on the packaging don't say "Complete and Balanced," and only list a few nutritional claims in very small print at the bottom. What the packaging *does* say is much more impressive to a trained eye than the previous brand example. It has a "Regional Ingredients Delivered Fresh" seal; it stipulates that the food source animals were "free-run" (similar to free-range) or "wild-caught"; it specifically states that the food is a single-grain formula (in this case, "steel-cut oats" and "oat flakes," both "oats," clearly defined and identified); it includes the words "never frozen" and "no preservatives"; and the food animals are clearly identified without the shopper even having to turn the bag around to look at the ingredients—in this case, they are "Free-Run Cobb Chicken, Whole Eggs, Wild-Caught Flounder, and Fruits and Vegetables." Note also that the bag identifies *precisely* the farms these animals, fruits, and vegetables were raised or grown in, and pinpoints the geographical regions where these farms are located. This second brand example does not have to entice the buyer with corny photos of happy, shiny dogs and slogans about man's best friend. To the *untrained eye*, this bag is underwhelming and falls short of inspiring immediate excitement for the buyer because of the lack of stimulating imagery. To one who has no intention of being hoodwinked by such marketing schemes, Good Guy's Recipe Kibble bypasses all that nonsense, allowing its concerns for your pet's welfare to speak for themselves in precise identification of central ingredients.

Now, let's compare the ingredients of Yum Yum's Poison Chow against Good Guy's Recipe Kibble. Note that pet food companies must list the ingredients by order of weight, so the higher up the item is on the list, the more weight that ingredient contributes to the total weight of the food. With *most* pet foods, the first five ingredients represent the majority of what the food contains, but this doesn't mean that the items at the end of the list are irrelevant, since many of them, even in tiny doses, over time, can cause health problems (such as dyes and preservatives). (Also note that the text in parentheses appears on the originals.)

Yum Yum's Poison Chow Ingredients

Beef by-product, high fructose corn syrup, soy grits, soy flour, water, wheat flour, corn syrup, calcium carbonate, phosphoric acid, salt, animal fat preserved with mixed tocopherals (form of vitamin E), sorbic acid (a preservative), calcium propionate (a preservative) DL-methionine, choline chloride, zinc sulfate, ferrous sulfate, ethoxyquin (a preservative), added color (Red 40), vitamin E supplement, manganese sulfate, niacin, vitamin A supplement, calcium pantothenate, thiamine mononitrate, copper sulfate, riboflavin supplement, vitamin B-12 supplement, pyridoxine hydrochloride, folic acid, vitamin D-3 supplement, calcium iodate, biotin, menadione sodium bisulfite complex (source of vitamin K activity), sodium selenate.

Good Guy's Recipe Kibble Ingredients

Chicken meal, deboned chicken, whole potato, steel-cut oats, peas, whole egg, deboned flounder, sun-cured alfalfa, chicken fat (preserved with mixed tocopherals), oat flakes, chicken liver, chicken liver oil, herring oil, pea fiber, whole apples, whole pears, sweet potato, pumpkin, butternut squash, parsnips, carrots, spinach, cranberries, blueberries, kelp, chicory root, juniper berries, angelica root, marigold flowers, sweet fennel, peppermint leaf, lavender, rosemary, vitamin A supplement, vitamin D3 supplement, vitamin E supplement, niacin, riboflavin, folic acid, biotin, vitamin B12 supplement, zinc proteinate, iron proteinate, manganese proteinate, copper proteinate, selenium yeast, dried Enterococcus faecium fermentation product. (Just under this list it says, "[This brand and recipe] is formulated to meet the nutritional levels established by the AAFCO dog food nutrient profiles for all life stages," showing the buyer that the producer has adhered to the high standards of AAFCO.)

Yum Yum's Poison Chow Comments

At this point in the book, the reader has likely noticed the very first nose-wrinkler in Yum Yum's Poison Chow. Beef by-product, the first item on the list, means various chopped-up pieces of cows. We don't know where the cows come from; what they were fed; how long they were dead, bloated, or both, before they were processed; what diseases they may have had; how many maggots rode in with them; how long and at what temperatures they were cooked during the rendering process; what other chemicals were added to the raw mix at the plant; and how much meat was still on them when they were processed, or whether the majority of that processing lot was a bunch of hooves and bones and brains. Whew!… That is *quite a lot* of information we *don't* have regarding the main ingredient!

The second item on the label is high fructose corn syrup. Aw, shucks, guys…you shouldn't have. No, really, you *shouldn't have.* There is absolutely nothing healthy about this sweetener for dogs, cats, humans, etc., and it's especially offensive that it's the second ingredient listed. (See previous chapter for several health concerns related to this and other sweeteners.)

Now, from the third ingredient on, nearly all of the terms are confusing, hard to pronounce, and extremely unfamiliar to the general public. It's not terribly inaccurate to say that only a scientist would know what this food actually has in it—and anytime a label is *that* complicated, you can assume the company is hiding a lot of terror under all that long-winded and garish wordiness that they know in advance the buyer won't understand.

We will not take the time here to visit each ingredient and its effect on dog biology (although there are some additional protein notes within the following pages), as we have already spent a good portion of the book doing just that. It should be noted, however, that several of these ingredients (such as Red No. 40 and ethoxyquin, just to name two that the reader will recognize from the previous chapter) refer to artificial preservatives and dyes that are very harmful and concerning.

Good Guy's Recipe Kibble Comments

The first two ingredients listed, "chicken meal" and "deboned chicken," are reassuring. Chicken meal, unlike chicken by-product meal, refers to clean flesh and skin (sometimes including bones), and is free of feathers, feet, heads (which means free of beaks and brains also), and entrails. Deboned chicken has a similar meaning, but without bones. We know from elsewhere on the Good Guy's Recipe Kibble packaging exactly what farm these chickens came from and how they were raised, so there is no ambiguity as to the quality of the source.

Other protein sources (whole egg and deboned flounder) are listed very high up on the label, and with the same respect to the origin of the source.

The only preservative listed in this label is mixed tocopherals. "Tocopherols are a family of vitamin E compounds naturally found in vegetable oils, nuts, fish and leafy green vegetables. The nutritional benefits of Vitamin E (d-alpha-tocopherol) and its importance as a daily part of the human diet have been well documented."[122] This is how Good Guy's Recipe Kibble can maintain that it is free of preservatives, because this ingredient, only used to preserve the oils of animal fats, is natural, and it is added to the animal fats, not to the food, itself. No preservative is added directly to this food.

Like the meats in this food, all fruits and vegetables are grown locally, with the farm in question named specifically.

Lastly, almost all of these ingredients are easy terms that clearly identify meats, fruits, and vegetables largely known by

the general public. All ingredients of major nutritional importance are listed first.

Yum Yum's Poison Chow "Protein" versus Good Guy's Recipe Kibble Protein

Before any erroneous assumptions are made regarding the
protein content of Yum Yum's Poison Chow in comparison to
the Good Guy's Recipe Kibble, the reader must be reminded
of one great truth: Protein can be found in many places, but
that doesn't mean that it's always from a good source. When
you view the "Guaranteed Analysis" of a cat or dog food label,
the proteins (as well as fats and fibers) are listed by percentage.
A person may be intrigued when a poor brand lists a higher
protein percentage than a better brand. (In this instance, the
"crude protein" is higher in the bag of Good Guy's Recipe
Kibble than it is in Yum Yum's Poison Chow, but that is not
always the case, and it can be misleading.) But getting to the
bottom of this mystery involves two things: 1) consideration
of the protein content sources, and 2) a simple mathematical
equation.

Sources: Earlier in this book, we mentioned that *hair* contains proteins. Leather does, too. Assuming that a bowl full of
leather chunks and hair is not the kind of protein you want to
provide your animal, then pay careful attention to where the
protein is coming from. If a brand doesn't list the origins, as
many do not, we can assume there's a lot of non-meat related
protein in the food. To avoid this, stick with a brand like
Good Guy's Recipe Kibble that lists identifiable meat sources

as the first item on the list (and preferably several other protein sources very early on), and which tells exactly where the ingredients come from.

A simple mathematical equation: If you're like these authors, then you hate math, and you immediately get discouraged when you hear the word. Don't distress…this one is easy. In order to figure the protein percentage within the food, you have to extract (or minus out) the moisture factor. When a food lists the percentage of proteins, fats, and fiber, it does *not* take into consideration the amount of water in the food. The "crude protein" as listed in the "Guaranteed Analysis" section of the label is based on the food as it rests within the bag or can. From one food to another, the moisture/water content differs, from as low as 6 percent to as high as 80 percent, so in order to compare one food's protein percentage to another, you have to convert both bags to "dry matter basis" (the mixture of the food without the water).

As an example, wet canned food is *much* higher in moisture than dry kibble. Mathematically zapping the moisture content (water) out of the canned food will give you the "dry matter basis," from which you can derive a more accurate count of the provided proteins. This will help buyers compare one protein claim to the next, and it's especially important when considering a change from wet food to dry food, or vise versa. (Again, don't fret. This is easy math. Stick with us.)

Starting with 100 percent, subtract the moisture rating (found in the analysis section of the label). Using Good Guy's Recipe Kibble as an example, we see "10 %" listed as the *maximum* amount of moisture. Take the whole food (100 percent) and subtract the moisture content (10 percent) and you get the following easy equation:

100 - 10 = 90

Therefore, 90 percent of the food is "dry matter," once the moisture is subtracted out.

Now, divide the percentage of protein content by the dry matter content. The "crude protein" listed on Good Guy's Recipe Kibble is 28 percent. So take 28 percent and divide it by 90 percent. If, like these authors, you can't do this in your head and you don't have a percentage calculator nearby, simply Google it ("28 % divided by 90 %" in the search field). This provides the following simple equation:

28% / 90% = 31%

Thus, in Good Guy's Recipe Kibble, 31 percent of the food content is protein. And, since this brand has efficiently declared where the protein is coming from, we have a much clearer picture of what this 31 percent is made up of.

In Yum Yum's Poison Chow, doing the same math delivers the following results:

100 percent of the whole food, minus 33 percent moisture, equals 67 percent dry matter (100 - 33 = 67).

18 percent of the crude protein content, divided by 67 percent dry matter, equals 26 percent protein content after moisture is removed (18% / 67% = 26%).

And, since this brand has *not* efficiently declared where the proteins are sourced, we have no idea what that 26 percent of protein includes.

So if a shopper were to compare the bags in a store, Yum Yum's Poison Chow would list 18 percent protein, and Good Guy's Recipe Kibble would list 28 percent protein, as it appears on the analysis portion of the label. Once calculated down to only dry matter, these numbers now become 31 percent and 26 percent. However, let's use another product by Yum Yum's to drive home the importance of this math for the label-comparing shopper. In Yum Yum's Poison Gravy-Giblets-In-A-Can canned food, we see the crude protein is 7 percent. The moisture rating is 82 percent. Canned foods often have huge moisture ratings compared to dry foods. Here's the math:

100 percent of the whole food, minus 82 percent moisture, equals 18 percent dry matter (100 - 82 = 18).

7 percent of the crude protein content, divided by 18 percent dry matter, equals 39 percent protein content after moisture is removed (7% / 18% = 39%).

Considering a canned food item, the protein content jumps from a tiny 7 percent all the way to almost 40 percent! That's quite a leap. Since so many pet owners are feeding their animals from a can, it is necessary that they understand how much of that can is water or fluids, and how much protein exists in the remaining mixture, in order to compare brands.

Note that this math is the same when determining the fats

and fiber, so we do not need to revisit this equation for those other factors here.

And Now, Ladies and Gentlemen, the True Story of the "Sweater Dog"

As a final thought on our comparison between Yum Yum's Poison Chow and Good Guy's Recipe Kibble, these authors would like to share a quick story.

A couple of years ago, one of Joe's closer acquaintances, Shane, had a twelve-year-old Chihuahua-Maltese mix named Cookie suffering severely from skin problems. Shane has had a lot of money since his career in computer technology was established. He lives in pricey homes, lounges on ornate furniture, and travels frequently. On one visit to Shane's home, Joe noticed Cookie was wearing a sweater. What would have normally been a cute scene of a precious family pet in an adorable outfit became immediately concerning when Joe observed the dog rubbing against everything in the home, itching, scratching, and scraping himself raw all over his coat, to the point that huge patches of his fur had been replaced by bloody, scabby sores open to infection. The sweater, Shane told Joe, was not for looks, but was a means to shield Cookie from doing additional harm to himself. The dog just didn't look well. He had droopy eyes and slow, lethargic movements.

At one point during his visit, Joe saw a bag of dog food and noted that the brand Shane had been giving Cookie was the same brand as that which we have been calling Yum Yum's Poison Chow. As a seasoned dog behavior consultant, Joe had identified these symptoms many times from his clients' dogs prior, and was highly suspicious that the food was the cause of the issues.

It wasn't that Shane didn't feel that Cookie deserved a better diet. His willingness to spend money on his dog as a part of the family had been proven numerous times when he had taken his pet to the vet and paid for exams and bloodwork in an attempt to get to the bottom of what was causing Cookie's condition, which Shane's veterinarian ultimately determined was a "mysterious allergy to something." Treatments at such visits, according to Shane's memory, included oral antibiotics to fight periodic yeast infections and a pharmaceutical topical ointment to soothe the itching and promote hair growth. *Not one time* in any of Shane's visits to the veterinarian was food or diet mentioned as a possible factor. In fact, the vet explained to Shane that, as a dog approaches his later years, these things can be expected. Shane loved his dog, and would have happily spent whatever money it took to improve Cookie's life. The reason Shane was feeding his dog Yum Yum's Poison Chow was simply because, like many consumers, he didn't know which brand to choose from all the misleading competition on the market, and since just about all of them make similar grand claims on their packaging, he had chosen the one that appealed to his *eyes* the most. His decision for Yum Yum's Poison Chow was not based on selfishness, but on being unaware of the secrets behind the pet food industry's marketing tactics. He, like many, assumed that someone out there was ensuring that the industry practiced healthy standards.

Joe didn't want to embarrass his friend, but he felt it was

his duty to say something, so he suggested a change in the dog's diet. Shane willingly agreed to try something new, and was very excited about the possibility that the solution to Cookie's maladies might be as simple as switching dog food. It seemed too good to be true that with all that complicated bloodwork, ointments, and medicines, Yum Yum's Poison Chow would be the easily correctable culprit. Joe and Shane discussed introducing new food, one much like Good Guy's Recipe Kibble, but grain-free.

Within one month of the switch, the itching and endless rubbing stopped, the sweater came off, and the dog's overall health had improved dramatically. Cookie has been in great health ever since.

Shane now spends less money on Cookie than he did before. Although the food is more expensive up front (but portions are much smaller, offsetting that cost over time), the vet bills and medical treatments are over. Buying the worst and cheapest foods for a pet may cost more in the long run, and the benefits of staying away from Yum Yum's Poison Chow are compelling and immediate.

Label Example Conclusion

This is just one example of comparison, based on only *two* available store-bought foods. One of them delights in fancy, flashy photos and claims on the bag (some of which are ridiculous, such as "Vitamins and Minerals," which would be included in any commercial pet food anyway, which is like a spaghetti sauce company claiming that *their* sauce "contains tomatoes" [oh my goodness...]), but some digging and comparison reveal that the company doesn't give a hoot about good nutrition. Not only are the ingredients they provide and in the order they are provided suspect of containing little nutritional value, their food presents a lot of potential harm to your animal. The other company doesn't rely on flashy packaging, as their food is just about as close as you can get to optimal health standards in the form of dry kibble available in chain stores, and the claims they do list on the packaging are backed up with evidence of transparency and accountability amidst the claims (such as alerting the buyer to the exact location of where all meats/vegetables are raised/grown). They have nothing to hide. Pet owners buying this brand will be able to make educated decisions for their pets instead of relying on company claims that either have no relevance or can hardly be proven. *This* is the kind of pet food that you want to purchase when you're out shopping and reading pet food labels.

The night before writing this chapter, these authors did a little field research. Going to see what was readily available for pets at the largest local supermarket, equipped with a camera, we raked through the aisles thoroughly. We considered every food label, both dry and canned, for both dogs and cats. We took pictures of many of the labels in order to refer to them later on for study and open-minded comparison. We actually *wanted* to find at least one brand of pet food in this major supermarket that compared to Good Guy's Recipe Kibble. Doing so would prove that the industry is progressing toward making healthier options available more conveniently than specialty stores. A few brands were certainly more promising than others, listing identified food animal sources as the first ingredient, as well as many clear and precise fruits and vegetables, but alas, by-products were contained in almost all of them, and when by-products weren't the issue, we had no way of knowing where the company had obtained the food animals. There wasn't one brand—*not one*—that didn't claim extreme health benefits for pets, and almost all stated the food was "complete and balanced." This was *not* a holistic health food store or a pet store, but the variety was probably at least double or triple what you would expect to find in a pet store, holistic or otherwise. Of every brand we searched, all claiming signs and wonders, we did not find *one* pet food we would recommend.

With that said, there were a few pluses to our little field trip. Of the hundreds of foods there, a few were new to the pet food department. One label followed all the same approaches to transparency and labeling as Good Guy's Recipe Kibble except for one major deal-breaker: Though the label on the bag did list some ingredients that would appear attractive up front, like identified meat sources, the purchaser would have no idea where any of the food animals had been raised. For all we know, the source animals had been raised in China and pumped with hormones before being butchered and sent to a secondary processing facility where preservatives were added to the meat before they were then sent to the pet food company. If dangerous chemicals or additives *can* be hidden, they will be. If a company has nothing to hide, it won't hide anything, including the origins of the sources used. (Note, however, that the presence of newer, more transparent brands is a good sign.)

If you're not finding what you're looking for at your major

supermarket, stop looking there. It's likely it is not focused on pet health, but on stocking the products that most closely match the demands of the store's clientele. If you wish to switch to a pet food that is like the Good Guy's Recipe Kibble example, try shopping at a store where the product *also* matches the demand of the clientele. A pet store specializing in holistic health for animals has a far better chance of carrying a healthy product, because it's what the customers are going there for in the first place. Common sense.

(Note: This example was made using dry kibble. However, see what Dr. Jean Hofve has to say about dry food versus canned food in the section of this book entitled "Interview with a Holistic Veterinarian.")

Pet Food Recalls and Bad News

Once you've found a store-bought food that you feel best suits your pet, check one additional issue before investing money into that brand: Find out whether there have been any associated recalls. If the food you are considering has never been recalled in the history of the company, that's a good sign. If there *has* been a recall, look it up and see what it was related to, when it happened, what animals were affected by it, and whether sufficient measures were taken to permanently correct the problem. The brand that we referred to in previous pages as Good Guy's Recipe Kibble has never experienced a recall.

Moreover, you should double check to see if the brand you are considering has ever been mentioned in major media for any controversial reason.

Take Blue Buffalo (a real company name) as one example. Since awareness has been growing among pet owners of the contaminant nature of by-products and the health issues associated with them, Blue Buffalo responded with very strong claims that its pet foods did not contain by-product meal. An estimated $50 million was spent promoting the by-product-free pet foods.[123] The company's advertising was so powerful and convincing that many shoppers switched to that brand and, for a time, they apparently felt secure in their purchases, even though they had to pay a hefty price for the food. However, Blue Buffalo made a mistake by advertising that other leading pet food brands were "misleading consumers"—and some competing pet food brands didn't take that sitting down.

Purina (also a real company name) launched its own independent lab studies on Blue Buffalo's food. In May of 2014, Purina filed a lawsuit against Blue Buffalo "for false advertising, disparagement and unjust enrichment."[124] In addition to Purina's complaints about its competitor's food containing *by-product meal*, egg shells, feathers, and harmful artificial preservatives, some of Blue Buffalo's "grain-free" recipes were shown to contain rice hulls. The result?

> The lawsuit follows a March 2014 decision of the National Advertising Division (NAD) of the Council of Better Business Bureaus, which found that Blue Buffalo is engaging in misleading advertising practices with respect to its claims about competing products. The NAD decision recommended that Blue Buffalo correct its television ad campaigns by removing all of

its allegations that Blue Buffalo's competitors are misleading consumers.[125]

The following September, Purina amended its complaint against Blue Buffalo to include further false advertising in association with cat litter and dog treats.

Finally, one year to the day after Purina had filed the initial lawsuit: "Blue Buffalo admitted the truth in court yesterday: A 'substantial' and 'material' portion of Blue Buffalo pet food sold over the past several years contained poultry by-product meal, despite pervasive advertising claims to the contrary."[126]

This was the *second time* that Blue Buffalo was linked with lies surrounding its ingredients. Prior to 2007, Blue Buffalo had claimed that its food did not contain melamine, "an industrial chemical traced to Chinese suppliers."[127] However, in 2007, Blue Buffalo was among many major brands (also including Purina) that faced a recall because of melamine contamination. In response to this newly found evidence, Blue Buffalo claimed that they had been lied to by their suppliers. In 2015, when they admitted that their food contained by-products, egg shells, preservatives, feathers, and grains (in the grain-free recipes) as a result of the *Purina v. Blue Buffalo* case, they claimed that they had been lied to by their suppliers.

This is a great example of the kind of deception that can happen in the pet food industry—the difference between Blue Buffalo and all other major liars being the simple fact that they got caught. Whether the deception occurred at the industry/marketing level (Blue Buffalo intentionally keeping this information from the public) or from the supply level (Blue Buffalo was hoodwinked by manufacturing contract suppliers and had no way of knowing their food contained by-products), the deception still carried through to the shopping carts of pet owners who were none the wiser and, therefore, to the pets who had feathers and egg shells for breakfast. (If there is any truth to Blue Buffalo's claims that the suppliers were at fault, these authors still wish to point out a very important caveat: *It is Blue Buffalo's responsibility to know what is going into their food. An audit of their supply chain would have revealed this.* Thus, the idea that Blue Buffalo was being lied to still points to the company as the guilty party for this deception by negligent practice. Any responsible food manufacturers will take necessary steps to find out what goods they are securing for their practice, and maintaining the quality of those sources.)

As of May 2015, only two months ago at the time of this writing, "Blue Buffalo still has not informed consumers of the presence of poultry by-product meal in Blue Buffalo pet food, refuses to accept responsibility for the product it sold, and is instead blaming its suppliers."[128]

But the study of this case between Purina and Blue Buffalo also reveals another interesting backtrack to Purina's own dirt. A class-action lawsuit was filed against Purina in association with illnesses and deaths in dogs as a result of mycotoxin poisoning in February of this year (2015).[129] Mycotoxin, as discussed earlier in this book, are toxins created by moldy grains. Purina's response to this lawsuit? The grains used in their foods are FDA approved. (Technically, this is true. The FDA allows for cheap grains—that which may contain mold and, therefore, mycotoxins—to be used in pet foods.) The

FDA has not issued a warning for Purina's affected foods, nor do they have any comment on the lawsuit.[130]

This, also, is *not* the only time that Purina's name has been dragged through the mud because of sick animals and widely covered scandals. (Although, it doesn't take big news to alert a pet owner of Purina's low nutrition standards. Many of their products, if not all, list whole grain corn, meat and bone meal, and corn gluten meal, among other useless items, as the first ingredients on their food labels. If pet owners are using the methods taught in the previous pages to weed out the poor choices from the better choices, they will see immediately that Purina is not as ideal as advertised.)

If you are considering a store-bought food, do a Google search to see what the producer's reputation has been in the industry and media, as well as any recalls associated with the company. Be informed.

Also *please note*, Dr. Jean Hofve has incredible insight on selecting commercial brands. Although she believes the home-prepared diet to be the absolute best method (and many holistic veterinarians agree), she understands that some pet owners may have to rely on a store-bought food under some circumstances. She provides additional valuable information on the selection process, which can be read at her website,[131] as well as in the "Interview with a Holistic Veterinarian" section of this book.

Chapter Six

Approaching Medicine

Medicine is not only a science; it is also an art. It does not consist of compounding pills and plasters; it deals with the very processes of life, which must be understood before they may be guided.
—Paracelsus[132]

As said earlier in the book, if veterinarians didn't sincerely wish to help animals, they wouldn't be in the field of animal care in the first place. For the most part, we can assume that *many* veterinarians are well meaning and genuine people who find extreme satisfaction in giving your pet the best possible care.

As we wind down this book, which focuses almost entirely on the pet food industry, there is one important point these authors feel must be made. There are also "bad guys" in the pet medicine industry. This is not to say that veterinarians are the bad guys, but that a score of treatments are available for your pet that can also present serious dangers. This is true in the veterinarian's office, just as it is true within the world of human medicine. Sometimes we have no choice but to treat a person or a pet with these products and drugs, because the consequences of nontreatment outweigh the potential risks of the drug.

However, when the health-related need is not immediate or serious, and holistic methods abound to treat the same condition just as effectively, why would we place our pets at risk if we don't have to? This question especially applies on a consumer level. Many at-home care products on the shelves of pet stores contain unnecessary and potentially toxic ingredients. And for a majority of those products, there is an alternative method of at-home care products that can either be purchased from a holistically minded specialty store (in person or online) or that can be made from standard, household items.

We will not visit that entire list here, as there are hundreds of options, and in a book of this length, trying to include them all would be space prohibitive. Just as a quick example, as a basis of comparison, let's take a look at one of the most popular at-home care products within the pet business.

Flea and Tick Treatments as One Example

How would you respond if you took your flea- or tick-infested cat or dog to a veterinarian, and the treatment was to pull out a can of bug spray and start spraying it all over your pet? Some might react with trust, assuming that the professionals know what they are doing, but many pet owners would be skeptical. Covering an animal in a cloud of toxic or deadly pesticides is not what many of us would accept without some very convincing statement of reassurance. And even then, we would likely return home and do some digging online to see if this treatment was, in fact, a regular practice. It would be a shock. No?

And yet, each time we buy almost any commercial flea or tick collars, sprays, powders, or some shampoos, we are essentially doing the same thing: subjecting our pets to dangerous chemicals.

The way that many of these products work, unbeknownst to the general public, is rather disturbing. Labels frequently warn against skin contact (especially regarding pregnant women), and state that consumers should keep out of the reach of children. The labels also feature instructions to wash hands immediately after use, etc., but how does that add up? Placing these harmful chemicals directly on your animal's coat and skin causes many of the substances to be absorbed by the skin and make their way into the bloodstream. That sounds like a "poison the dog to poison the pest" approach, and that can't possibly be how it works, right? But perhaps it is… Many stories nationwide have surfaced that tell of pets immediately reacting to flea and tick treatments with conditions like seizures, vomiting, diarrhea, and trouble breathing. If *you* shouldn't get these chemicals on your skin, why should we assume it's safe for our other mammal friends? If *you* shouldn't put the pesticides in your mouth, why would it be safe for our pets to lick their coats after we have dosed them with it?

Unnatural Treatments

You have probably heard of "spot-on" treatments—little vials of the "medicine" packaged within small boxes, and they are usually very expensive. The leading brands are Frontline, Frontline Plus, Advantage, K9 Advantix II, PetArmor, Defend, Zodiac, Biospot, and ProMeris. Flea and tick collars—with leading brands including Zodiac, Sergeants, Pet Agree, Longlife, and Hartz—are among the most popular treatments. These rubbery collars emit a cloud of toxins around your pet at all times for the life of the chemical, presenting a danger to your pet as well as to yourself when you snuggle up against them. If the collars come loose, there's an additional risk that cats and dogs might gnaw on the chewy material and orally ingest the toxins.

Some of the leading active ingredients in these products include imidacloprid, fipronil, permethrin, pyrethrin, phenothrin, methoprene, amitraz, and pyriproxyfen. Several of these work by affecting the insects' nervous system, causing paralysis and eventually death (a neurotoxin to the insect). When applied to an animal's skin (usually in once-a-month doses), the oils from the flea treatment mixture adhere to the hair follicles of the animal, and the chemicals release slowly over time. Other ingredients in this list are "juvenile hormone analogs," which prevent larvae from reaching adulthood and, thus, from reproducing. Let's take a brief look at a few of these.

Imidacloprid:[133] Not active against ticks (however, note that many flea and tick products contain both imidacloprid and permethrin, the latter of which is effective against ticks). It should noted that imidacloprid *has not been* one of the most dangerous active ingredients for cat and dog flea treatments, as they have handled it well historically. However, the ingredient *has been* tested on mice, rats, and dogs, and in some higher doses,

prolonged lower doses (excess use over time), as well as accidental mishandling (especially upon oral entrance to the body, so
watch those "coat-licker" pets), can be dangerous, according to
lab testing. In addition, smaller animals have shown a greater
likelihood of having adverse reactions. Issues associated with this
ingredient in mammals (which includes pet owners, if they are
not careful when administering the treatment) include:

- Fatigue or lethargy
- Convulsions, seizures, or tremors
- Difficulty breathing
- Painful cramps
- Incoordination
- Transient growth retardation, developmental
  retardation, and reproductive toxicity
- Degenerative changes in the testes, bone marrow,
  pancreas, and thymus
- Cardiovascular affects
- Hematological affects
- Complications to the liver and thyroid
- Weight loss
- Neurobehavioral deficits (in rats and rabbits)
- Vomiting
- Excessive drooling
- Skin reactions
- Eye irritation
- Not approved for use on livestock in most countries
  (including the US)
- There is no antidote for imidacloprid poisening

Permethrin:[134] Permethrin is not completely safe for dogs *or* cats, but it is well known to be *very toxic to cats*! Two things should be kept in mind about this product: 1) A pet owner should *never* give canine flea or tick treatment to a cat, and 2) a pet owner should *never* give a flea or tick treatment containing permethrin to a dog that lives in close proximity to cats. In cats, permethrin poisoning is usually fatal (*many cats have died from being given permethrin*), and can cause convulsions, hyperaesthesia, hyperthermia (elevated body temperature), hypersalivation (excessive drooling), and loss of balance. These symptoms usually occur in smaller animal, and within hours of the dose. As with imidacloprid, higher doses and prolonged or excessive exposure are the most threatening to the animal, but many pet owners have reported adverse effects themselves after administering the treatment. Symptoms related to permethrin poisoning in animals can include:

- Potential of death
- Tremors
- Hypersalivation (excessive drooling)
- Lack of appetite
- Vomiting
- Diarrhea
- Incoordination
- Disorientation
- Hyperactivity
- Depression
- Difficulty breathing
- Seizures

- Ear flicking
- Paw shaking
- Contractions/twitching of the skin
- Skin redness or irritation/itching

Amitraz:[135] This ingredient is also incredibly toxic for cats (as well as for horses). Adverse reactions are caused by the alpha-adrenergic agonist activity. Symptoms associated with amitraz include:

- Potential of death
- Low blood pressure
- Decreased body temperature
- Elevation of blood glucose
- Dilated pupils
- Slowed heart rate
- Slowed intestinal rate
- Ataxia (loss of control over body movements)
- Vasoconstriction (the narrowing of blood vessels)
- Vomiting
- Diarrhea
- Seizures
- Sedation (and prolonged sedation)
- Dry skin
- Dry coat

We will not continue to break down the dangers behind every chemical found in flea and tick treatments. As a general rule, if a medicine is not natural, and an equally effective natural method is available alternatively, you should always do what is natural.

Natural Treatments

Not only are these natural treatments much healthier for your pet, but many of them are pleasant for the pet owner as well, and they involve insect-repelling tactics that have been used for centuries.

Wash bedding as frequently as the infestation requires: One of the most common hang-out centers for fleas is in the pet's bedding. The following methods will have a lesser chance of working if your cat or dog immediately returns to a flea-infested bed.

Natural flea and tick treatments from a store: Available in many holistic pet stores, natural flea and tick treatments aren't very hard to find. If you are a busy person, and some of the methods below sound too time-consuming or repetitive, do a little digging. Many online pet product stores carry insect-repelling products that work just as efficiently as the major market treatments, and they have very pleasant scents.

Bathing: Oh-so-many holistic veterinarians wonder why the majority of pet owners don't take their pets straight to the bathtub when they show signs of flea infestation. Generally speaking, soap and water kills fleas. But when the season produces a stronger fleet of pests, there are a few things you can add to a routine bath that will zap them. First, use real soaps such as like castile soap (and be sure to dilute, as the soaps are highly concentrated), which cause insects to die from dehydration as a result of cell-membrane interference. (Again, avoid pesticide-based shampoos. Remember not to bathe pets too often, especially cats. Over-bathing strips the skin and coat of natural oils. Cats are self-bathers, so if this method doesn't work, try another method.)

Spray: A well-known remedy for fleas that works well for dogs and cats (and does not change pH levels) is home-made apple cider vinegar spray. Some recipes suggest diluting with water and others do not, depending on the size of the animal and whether it is being applied to a dog or a cat. Because these authors do not know the size and species of your pet, we cannot suggest an exact recipe, but it should be stated that the only difference in the recipes would be for the purposes of varying strength. Apple cider vinegar is a perfectly safe alternative to the dangers of chemically enhanced flea treatments.

Garlic: Fleas don't like garlic. Whether you are following the home-prepared, raw, or store-bought diet methods, add a pinch of fresh garlic to your pet's bowl. Not only will this deter fleas, it also discourages worms and other parasites.

Cedar oil and cedarcide: One caveat, readers. The verdict is still out on whether cedar oil can be used on cats, because essential oils are often highly toxic to cats. (Dogs, however, shouldn't be a problem.) From one veterinarian to another, the responses on this are conflicting, as some say the store-bought oil in the form we normally have access to is dangerous, and others say it's perfectly safe. However, certain species of cedar trees contain an oil that is said *not* to be an issue for cats at all—Wondercide, for example. On its website, Wondercide states that its cedar oil is a "modified Eastern Red Cedar oil that is properly diluted with a hydrated silica carrier oil at a 90% ratio. It is not known to be harmful to cats or kittens, since **it does not contain phenols, or phenolic compounds**, which occur naturally in many essential oils."[136] So if you wish to try this method on your cat, you may not be as out of luck as some sources claim. To approach this method cautiously, consult your veterinarian if you are considering using cedar oil on your cat. If using it on a dog, applying it to the coat directly (avoiding the face, eyes, and nose, as it has a powerful, woodsy smell) will jumpstart the process of repelling fleas, and a homemade flea collar with the same ingredient will maintain the protection (for a longer period, at least). To avoid having to figure out a mixture for coat application (and to avoid the mess the oil can make), many stores sell it pre-mixed (visit CedarCide.com as an example). To make a collar, mix three to five drops of cedar oil with one to three tablespoons of water and dip the collar (or a bandana) in the mixture, then simply place the collar on around your dog's neck as usual. The scent is strong and can be overpowering, so the amount of oil you apply directly to the coat, and whether you should dilute it depends on the size of your dog. Some apply drops directly to the coat, and others dilute with water and use a spray bottle to apply to the treatment. Whether you make your own mixture or buy it pre-made, it is always important to remember that as water and oil don't mix, a good shaking up is always needed before application. As an added upkeep, placing cedar chips in your dog's bed (as many of them zip open) also helps keep the fleas from returning to your dog's favorite rest area.

Lemon: Natural lemon (but not the peel, as it contains

limonene, which is not always safe for pets) is a great deterrent for pests. Squeeze fresh lemon juice into a bath, mix it with water for a spray, or dip your pet's comb in it directly are all great ways to apply one of nature's best remedies for fleas.

Rose Geranium Oil: This oil is surprisingly effective against ticks, and it is safe for both dogs and humans (unless there is a specific allergy, which is rare). Many sources say that it is also safe for cats, but some claim otherwise (as many essential oils are not); still others say it depends on whether or not you are purchasing the correct oil, so, as always, double check with your veterinarian before applying to a feline. (It also happens to be used to enhance athletic performance, promote weight loss, and ease nerve pain in humans.[137]) There are two kinds of rose geranium oil: *Pelargonium capitatum xradens* and *Pelargonium graveolens*. *Pelargonium capitatum xradens* is the botanical name to look for, as it delivers better results. Because canines are especially sensitive to smell, don't overdo the application. The most highly recommended dosage for dogs is to apply one drop behind each shoulder blade and one drop at the base of the tail; for cats, apply one drop between shoulder blades and one drop at the base of the tail. Because this method is also safe for humans, and because many people have found this a simple way to repel pests on themselves during outdoor activities with their pets, human application of this method is as follows: one drop on each wrist, one drop on each ankle, one drop behind each knee, and one drop behind each ear (or one drop on the back of the neck).

In addition to all these methods above are at least twenty or thirty more that many claim are effective. We have only included the most popular ones here, but it is safe to assume that no pet owner should ever have to submit his or her pet to toxicity in order to battle pests. One thing to consider is this: Home remedies for pest control are not a one-and-done method. They require repeated applications and maintenance in order to ensure success. The good news is that many of them take just seconds to do—and your pet will thank you for it.

Keep in mind: In the same way that a person asks his or her physician about the safest and healthiest options for prevention and treatment of medical issues, pet owners should ask their vets educated questions regarding the safest and healthiest decisions to make about their animals' care. A little research makes for an all-around more efficient care procedure.

This doesn't just apply to addressing irregular symptoms that may pop up in your pet's behavior or physical condition, but to routine care as well. To illustrate the importance of knowing how to approach at-home products more safely, we used flea and tick treatments as an example. To illustrate the importance of preparing for a clinic visit, let's use vaccinations as an example.

Vaccines: One Example of Asking the Right Questions

If you know your pet's annual vaccinations are coming up, before you hand over your dog or cat willy-nilly to let the professionals do their job, it is prudent to dig a little deeper into the subject of vaccines so you can approach the office visit with questions that will lead to the most optimal care, as well as to avoid unnecessary treatment. Just a superficial search online will flood your computer screen with articles addressing the controversy of pet vaccination.

Anyone who has even briefly visited the subject of human vaccination will know that both professional and layperson opinions jump from "We're all gonna die without them" to "We're all gonna die because of them." It's practically impossible to find a solid position for or against giving our babies shots without educating ourselves first. The same is true for animals. Many believe vaccines are essential, and many believe they are useless. Some land in a central camp somewhere between these two extremes, suggesting that initial vaccinations are a must, but that subsequent shots only need to be given every seven years or so—never annually.

Research doesn't have to take long. Sometimes, a ten-minute skimming of readily available information is all you need to prepare for a clinic visit. As a case in point, these authors just typed in the words "vaccinations dangerous for pets" on a Google search. Links to hundreds of articles popped up, but let's focus on just the first three in the order in which they appeared in the search results. All are short enough to read quickly.

Here is an excerpt from the first, by Dr. Becker of Mercola's Healthy Pets Online:

The current canine vaccine schedule used by many veterinarians calls for annual immunizations for the following diseases:

- Rabies
- Parvovirus
- Distemper
- Adenovirus
- Parainfluenza
- Leptospirosis
- Coronavirus
- Hepatitis
- Lyme (borelia)
- Bortadella (kennel cough)

The annual schedule for cats includes vaccinations for:

- Rabies
- Feline leukemia (FeLV)
- Distemper
- Rhinotracheitis
- Calcivirus…

These entirely unscientific recommendations were introduced by the USDA and vaccine manufacturers over 20 years ago, and many veterinarians continue to follow them today despite mounting concerns about the health risks associated with over-vaccinating.[138]

From this article alone, we can assimilate the following questions:

- What is the pet being vaccinated for specifically?
- What are the risks associated with those vaccines?

- What are the risks associated with over-vaccinating or annual vaccines?
- What are the dangers of choosing not to vaccinate?

In the second article that popped up in our search, also by Mercola's Healthy Pets Online, we read the following:

Vaccinosis…is a problem only holistic veterinarians seem willing to acknowledge. It is a reaction of a pet's body to vaccines that have been injected… These are chronic reactions to not only the altered virus contained in the vaccine, but also to the chemicals, adjuvants, and other components of tissue culture cell lines—as well as possible genetic changes—that can be induced by vaccines.[139]

From this article, we can add the following questions to our list:

- What is "vaccinosis"?
- Have any of the other animals you have treated at this clinic shown signs of this?
- What signs should I be watching for in my cat or dog that would point to vaccinosis, and what is the follow-up treatment of these symptoms?
- Are there certain vaccines we can skip at this time to help avoid this?

In the third article that appeared, published by HolVet: Holistic Veterinary Services, we see mention of law requirements and appropriate dosage, which may be a very easy, but important, topic to address:

> Especially in the case of rabies vaccines, where boosters are *required by law*, it is important to minimize potential problems. Our practice is careful to administer a dose appropriate to the size of the animal—a Chihuahua does not need the same dose as a mastiff![140]

Thus, further questions materialize:

- Is choosing not to vaccinate even a choice, or does our county have laws requiring vaccination?
- If there *are* laws requiring vaccination, are some optional?
- When you administer the vaccine dose, do you consider the size of the dog? Or do you have a one-dose-fits-all model at this clinic?

Educating yourself before you visit a clinic can:

- Save your pet from potentially receiving unnecessary injections (which other veterinarians' articles refer to as incredibly toxic)
- Cut back on the costs of unnecessary treatments
- Save time during the visit because specific questions

are answered, instead of broader questions that require much more preliminary explanation

- Establish a mutual respect between pet owner and veterinarian
- Inform the veterinarian that he or she is working with a pet owner who will, in this visit as well as future visits, wish to approach the pet's treatment prudently and wisely

Whether the visit regards vaccines or symptoms requiring medical attention, a little bit of self-education and research prior to the visit goes a *long* way—and again, this can usually be accomplished in a very short time.

Respect Professionals in the Field

One final thought before we close this chapter. Whereas these authors always suggest asking questions and approaching a veterinarian with strong concern for the welfare of your pet, remember to always speak respectfully. Do not treat pet care professionals as if you know more than they do because you've read a book or two. Don't talk to them as if they are the enemy because their offices carry out certain treatments you disagree with. Sometimes a clinic operates under specific legal requirements (such as the rabies shot just mentioned), or its clinicians may have good reasons for conducting their treatments the way they do. If you are polite and armed with solid information, you will gain their respect, and that relationship will benefit everyone involved. On the other hand, if you talk down to them or come off as being defensive, you'll introduce tension and you may not inspire the professional to give your precious furry family member the best care.

In the end, if you suspect that a veterinarian does not have your pet's health in his or her best interest, there is no law against gracefully declining his or her assistance and finding another veterinarian who better suits your needs. But, above all, remember that the majority of the vet's time is spent trying to lend a helping hand to members of the animal kingdom, and that alone deserves great respect, whether or not the professional carries that torch precisely how a pet owner wishes him to.

Interview with a
Holistic Veterinarian

*No, feel free to ask any and all questions about [the pet food industry].
I just WISH more people knew about what was going on!*
—Dr. Jean Hofve, DVM[141]

In order to provide further insight on these subjects, these authors reached out to a holistic veterinarian. The following is an interview addressing many of the issues discussed within this book. Please note that some of the information provided in the following interview has been presented in previous chapters. For the sake of keeping the integrity of the original interview, we have kept Dr. Jean Hofve's responses intact.

Dr. Jean Hofve, what can you tell us about GMO in pet foods, and the effects that it has on the animals' welfare? Roundup is carcinogenic, and you've shared with us that somewhere around 90 percent of the corn used in pet foods is GMO corn sprayed with Roundup (and/or equivalent off-brands with the same chemicals). How does the toxicity of Roundup translate to the plant, and then to the animal ingesting the food? What are the generational implications of this in future litters?

Well, 95 percent of both corn and soy grown in the US is GMO, so unless it's organic (the other 5 percent) it is GMO. Pet food uses feed-grain corn, which is the worst.

Glyphosate (the active ingredient in Roundup) is taken up by the plant and distributed throughout the plant's tissues, including the fruit, vegetable, or seed.

Mercola.com and OrganicConsumers.org have a lot of good info on glyphosate, so I won't reinvent the wheel.

How can someone determine if there are GMOs in their pet food? Is that possible? Can the companies that claim to be GMO-free be trusted in this claim?

If it has nonorganic corn or soy, then it has GMOs.

Is there a source you trust and recommend that folks can use in finding good, easy-to-make, healthy recipes for cooking their own pet foods?

Yep! You can find this information on my website here: http://www.littlebigcat.com/nutrition/easy-homemade-diets-for-cats-and-dogs/. [Note that Dr. Hofve has written another incredibly helpful article regarding selecting store-bought foods here: http://www.littlebigcat.com/nutrition/selecting-a-good-commercial-pet-food/.]

What is the difference between independent rendering plants and captive rendering plants?

Independents take anything from any source. Did you see the *Dirty Jobs* episode about rendering? It's on YouTube. It currently costs $1.99. Watch it. That is an "independent" renderer. [This episode is also available on Amazon Instant Play, which is the source these authors used to view it.]

Captives are closely associated with a feedlot, slaughterhouse, etc. For instance, Tyson's chickens will all go to the same rendering plant, which only processes Tyson chickens.

We note that you had/have a friend who was an executive in a rendering company. What are some of the stories you've heard from him? Didn't you mention something about dead cows lying on the side of the road between pickups for weeks at a time?

Yes, for Darling International. Sadly, he died a few months after he first got in touch with me. What he told me was that it is *easy* for rendering plants to separate items, for instance, to *not* load the long-dead cows in the same vat as by-products fresh from the slaughterhouse and destined for dog food. But they don't.

Why are rendering companies so secretive?

Because it's a gross, filthy industry, and they don't want the public to get too interested in what they do. They were very unhappy with the revelations about what *can* go into pet food, and they pulled the curtain shut even tighter.

Why is it a good idea to get a product that has a meat source that is clearly named and identified as opposed to references of just "meat," generically?

"Meat" and "meat meal" can be from any one or a combination of four species: cows, sheep, goats, or pigs. "Meat and bone meal" (which is a single ingredient, not "meat" + "bone meal") can be from any mammalian species.

The upshot is that "meat" with a name probably comes from a captive rendering plant that is making a relatively pure product. This may not matter all that much unless/until your pet develops an allergy; and then you really need to know what's what, in order to avoid the allergen.

However, several studies have documented that there is a great deal of cross-contamination that happens, especially in OTC products. What is on the label has only a 60 percent chance of being accurate.

Can you clarify the differences between all the different by-product terminology? What's the difference between terms like "meat meal" and "chicken meal," etc?

"Meals" are rendered products and found mostly in dry food. Neither meat meal nor chicken meal (are supposed to) contain any by-products.

What do you have to say about vaccinations?

[As an answer to this question, Dr. Hofve directed us to one of her many helpful websites, where she discusses the issue at length: http://www.littlebigcat.com/health/vaccination/. We highly recommend all readers to take a look at her article prior to vaccinating any animal.]

What is the average life span of animals today, and how does that differ from the life span these animals should have? Are there more cancer-related deaths among dogs and cats today than in the past?

The average life span of a cat is between twelve to fifteen years. It is longer now than before, I believe mainly because more cats are kept indoors where they're not exposed to the many hazards of the world (see my article "Indoors or Outdoors?" here: http://www.littlebigcat.com/health/indoors-or-outdoors/). But it used to be fairly common to see cats in their twenties, and this is becoming much more rare.

In dogs, life span depends on size. Small dogs are similar to cats, but giant breeds (Irish Wolfhounds, Great Danes, etc.) live on average only seven to eight years before dying of heart disease or cancer.

Vets (and pet food companies and pharmaceutical companies) say that pets are living longer because of vaccines and commercial pet foods. However, I researched this extensively for our book *Paleo Dog* [available on Amazon; for more info see

Hofve's website at the following: http://www.paleodogbook.com/], and the average dog life span today is still the same as the average wolf life span (when free roaming is restricted). So, no real change in life span, but a much higher incidence of disease and cancer being seen in very young animals.

As a vet student, I saw a six-month-old Akita who had a terrible form of leukemia; the most optimistic prognosis was six months. (I was FURIOUS with the resident who talked these people into treating the dog, because the couple had a two-year-old. So the kid will have six months to get even more attached to a sick dog that's going to die anyway. Ack!) A friend's mare (who got every vaccine and dewormer we learned about in vet school) gave birth to a filly who was born with stomach cancer. Many breeds (golden retrievers and boxers especially) have a high incidence of lymphoma. Half of all dogs who are over the age of ten today will die of cancer. None of this was previously the case.

Life span is a very, very complicated issue affected by a host of influences: genetics, toxin exposure, vaccines, diet, stress… See my article, "Cancer Prevention and Treatment," at the following link: http://www.littlebigcat.com/?s=cancer.

What are some of the diseases that you've dealt with during your practice? Is there a story or two that stand out from the rest that reflect dietary responsibility of pet owners?

My favorite was a four-month-old kitten who had chronic diarrhea and had been treated with seven (SEVEN!) rounds of antibiotics. I put her on a raw meat diet, and by THE NEXT DAY the diarrhea cleared up and never came back.

Sadly, it cuts the other way, too. When our clinic was sold, the new owner stopped feeding raw meat to the clinic cats. The next time I saw Miss O'Neal, a beautiful seven-year old black and white long-haired cat, six months later, she looked awful. Her fur was dull and matted, and she had no energy. She died of cancer not long afterward.

In reading a food label, what might one look for in the first few listed ingredients?

I don't encourage just looking at the first few ingredients; it misses too much. If someone is willing to learn about that, they can learn to read the whole label. I most often find deal-breaker ingredients far down the list, like menadione [one of the listed ingredients in our Yum Yum's Poison Chow example above] and carrageenan [another harmful and cancer-causing ingredient found in pet foods].

What is this we hear about pet foods claiming to be "human-grade," as in, fit for human consumption?

Right now there is only ONE human-grade pet food manufacturer on the planet and that is The Honest Kitchen.

The rest are flat-out lying and making an illegal claim. The rule is: If you say human-grade, then every single ingredient AND the final product must be human-edible. *None* of them meet that standard. Even if they start with "human-grade" chicken, the minute that chicken leaves the slaughterhouse in an unsanitary, unrefrigerated truck, it is no longer human-edible. AAFCO is working on this issue, but slower than molasses in January.

What do you feed your own pets?

A combination of homemade raw, freeze-dried raw, and canned foods. They love kibble but I won't let them have it.

AAFCO's planning to meet in August to discuss their current regulation standards. I understand one of the concerns you have expressed to them for years regarding cross contamination is on their agenda to address as a result of your persistence. What do you hope will be the outcome of this?

They scheduled discussion on the fact that multiple studies have found massive cross-contamination and deliberate substitution of ingredients without a label change, so consumers cannot trust pet food labels to be truthful. I hope the outcome will be that industry takes this seriously and decides to quit screwing around! But, I doubt it.

In human medical care, many doctors treat symptoms instead of helping patients correct health concerns before they start. Is this the same for animal care? Why does the average veterinarian lack so much knowledge about the holistic approach to caring for animals, and how does that translate into so many poor medicine prescriptions/food recommendations?

Yes, but that's the $64,000 question! The simple answer is that medical and veterinary schools don't teach it. The why is more complex, but as they say, "follow the money." The pharmaceutical industry, the pet food industry, agribusiness, etc., want vets to stock and prescribe their products, and they have a lot of influence over veterinary education. The #1 veterinary nutrition textbook, for instance, is published by Hill's [a *very* popular pet food manufacturing company that surrounds its products with convincing claims on its packaging and in media; many holistic veterinarians find this food to be void of true nutritional value].

Joe Ardis, the central author behind this book, recently spoke with his vet regarding the many flea and tick collars/treatments releasing a harmful pesticide into the bloodstream, and that it is only when the flea/pest bites the animal that it is exposed to what kills it. (Joe wasn't trying to bait his vet into an awkward verbal exchange, but he was curious about what his professional response would be.) At Joe's remarks, the veterinarian nodded without surprise, and said, "Well, sure. It is a pesticide. We're treating pests." Just to be sure the vet had understood him, Joe explained that the dog or cat lives in a constant state of poisoning for the duration of the treatment, and that this couldn't possibly be healthy for the animal. The vet responded,

"Well, you know, we've been doing this for years, and it's just how we treat pets with fleas and ticks." Can you confirm that this form of treatment actually does poison the animal for the duration of the treatment? Can you recommend an alternative treatment such as cedar oil?

Theoretically, the poison is specific to insects and is not supposed to affect mammals. *However*, every flea/tick product registered with the EPA has caused illness and death in pets. Every single one of them.

We have been researching natural flea/tick remedies for cats and dogs, and although we have been able to find almost everything we're looking for online and in books, the jury is still out on a few items. Is the following oil (a natural tick repellant) safe for cats? Many say it is, but a few say it is not. Even more claim that geranium oil is safe for cats, but that is not an exact match. Your opinion on *Pelargonium capitatum xradens*, rose geranium oil?

I am not an herbalist, but I can tell you that a great many essential oils are highly toxic to cats. I checked the one source I have that you can't access through Google yourself, and found nothing specific on this oil.

I would be very concerned about using this or any essential oil directly on a cat, especially because oils are not only absorbed directly through skin, but the cat will also ingest a fair amount when grooming. Very few essential oils are safe for cats. See: http://www.littlebigcat.com/health/aromatherapy-and-essential-oils-for-pets/.

Cats are much more sensitive to essential oils than dogs, because their livers cannot metabolize them.

Natural flea/tick remedies don't work very well compared to drugs, but they are generally safer (for dogs). You still have to work hard at all the other aspects. The following is a link that will prove helpful to this issue: http://www.onlynaturalpet.com/holistic-healthcare-library/fleas-ticks/53/the-natural-approach-to-flea-control.aspx.

Why is dry dog food so much worse than wet dog food?

There are ten[142] reasons:

1. Ingredients: Dry food is typically made from rendered ingredients, such as chicken meal, poultry by–product meal, and meat and bone meal (MBM). Rendering starts with animal-source ingredients being fed into a massive grinder to reduce them to chunks. The resulting hodgepodge is boiled at high temperatures for hours or even days, turning everything to mush. Fat floats to the top and is skimmed off for other uses. The remainder is dried to a low-moisture, high protein powder suitable for use in dry foods.

Some rendered products are better—or worse—than others. Chicken meal, for instance, is likely to be relatively pure, because the rendering plant is usually associated with a slaughterhouse that processes only chickens. On the other end of the spectrum, MBM is the "dumping ground" of the nastiest raw ingredients.

Because all of this ends up as an amorphous brown powder, it's impossible to know what went into it. However, the U.S. Food and Drug Administration (FDA) found that dog foods containing MBM and/or "animal fat" (both rendered ingredients) were the most likely to contain pentobarbital, the primary drug used to euthanize animals.

In some dry foods, such as those found at grocery stores, discount stores, and large pet supply stores, even rendered meat is too costly to make the needed profit, so manufacturers substitute rendered by-product meals and/or vegetable proteins such as corn gluten meal, soybean meal, and plant protein concentrates to get the protein up to acceptable levels.

Other ingredients of the dough include carbohydrates, or starch (either grains or starchy vegetables), a vitamin-mineral premix, and water. Adult dogs and cats do not need any carbohydrates in their diet; all these starches do is provide calories. Because they aren't a natural part of our carnivorous pals' diets, most of those calories are quickly converted to fat. And then veterinarians wonder why we have a "pet obesity epidemic"!

2. Processing: To make dry food, whatever rendered high-protein meal is being used is mixed into a sticky, starchy dough that can be pressed through an extruder, which forms the kibble. The dough is forced by giant screws through a barrel and ultimately into tiny tubes that end in a shape, much like a cake decorator. The heat and pressure in the extruder are tremendous. As the compressed dough exits into the air, it passes through a whirling mass of sharp knives that cuts the pieces individually as they "pop" when they reach normal air pressure, creating the familiar shapes associated with each pet food brand.

While heat processing makes vegetables, fruits, and grains more digestible, it has the opposite effect on proteins. Not only are cooked proteins less digestible, but they can be distorted, or "denatured," by heating. These abnormal proteins may be a factor in the development of food allergies, as the immune system reacts to these unfamiliar and unnatural shapes.

Enzymes, special proteins that aid in thousands of chemical reactions in the body, are especially fragile, and are rapidly destroyed by heat, even at relatively low temperatures. The normal food enzymes that would help digest the food are destroyed by processing. This forces the pancreas to make up for those lost enzymes. Over time, the pancreas can become stressed and enlarged, and even get pushed into life-threatening pancreatitis.

3. Carbohydrates: Carbohydrates are molecules that contain carbon (C), hydrogen (H), and oxygen (O)—carbon and water (H_2O)—in other words, "hydrated carbon." The simplest carbohydrate is sugar; and all carbs are varying configurations of sugars. Fiber is a special type of carbohydrate made by plant cells to keep their cell walls rigid, allowing plants to grow upright from a relatively small base.

Dogs and cats are carnivores, meat-eaters. Their natural diet is high protein and high moisture. The carnivore's ideal diet is essentially the Atkins diet: lots of protein and fat, and a small amount of complex carbohydrates from vegetables.

Dogs (and humans) use carbs directly for energy by breaking them down to simple sugars. Sugars not needed for immediate energy, or to replenish glycogen stores in the liver and muscles, are turned into fat. This takes place through several biochemical pathways; but a major pathway used by most mammals (involving the enzyme glucokinase) is essentially absent in the cat. Cats are simply not built to process carbohydrates. Cats preferentially use protein and fat for energy, and these pathways are mandatory. Felines have very limited ability to process carbohydrates, and are "programmed" to turn carbs directly into fat.

Another disadvantage of carbohydrates is that they have a high glycemic index; this means that they raise blood sugar higher and faster than other nutrients. Increased blood sugar triggers the release of the hormone insulin from the pancreas. Insulin allows sugars to be absorbed into cells, where they can be used for fuel. Without insulin, no matter how fuel-starved cells may be, sugars stay in the bloodstream.

Heat processing increases the glycemic index of carbohydrates. Corn—a common ingredient of dry food—has a glycemic index similar to a chocolate bar. When dry food is available all the time, cats in particular will nibble at it fifteen to twenty times a day. This causes multiple sharp swings in blood sugar and requires the pancreas to secrete insulin each time. Over-secretion of insulin causes cells to down-regulate and become resistant to insulin. This is one reason why dry food is a major contributor to feline (Type II) diabetes.

4. Calories: It's currently estimated that about 50 percent of dogs and cats in the US are overweight, and many are seriously obese. Carrying extra weight isn't cute and cuddly—it will shorten your pet's life, create unnecessary discomfort, and will surely lead to one or more chronic diseases, such as diabetes, bladder and kidney disease, arthritis, liver failure, chronic gastrointestinal problems, poor immunity, and even cancer. You're not doing your pet any favors by giving in to those abnormal appetites, which are in most cases caused and perpetuated by dry food.

5. Dehydration: Obviously, dry food is dry. This is a big problem for cats, whose ancestors are desert-dwelling wild cats. They have passed on to our pets their super-efficient kidneys, which are designed to extract every last drop of moisture from prey animals. As a result, cats have a low thirst drive, and don't drink water until they are about 3 percent dehydrated— a dehydration level so serious that most veterinarians would consider giving intravenous fluids. Dogs have a higher thirst drive and will drink more readily, so they are less prone to dehydration.

Dehydration causes or contributes to many serious health issues, including urinary crystals and stones, bladder infections, FLUTD, constipation, and kidney disease.

6. Potential Contaminants: Given the types of things manufacturers put in pet food, such as pesticide-soaked grains and diseased, dead, and dying animals, it is not surprising that bad things sometimes happen. Ingredients used in pet food are often highly contaminated with a wide variety of toxic substances. Some of these are destroyed by processing, but others are not.

• *Bacteria & bacterial toxins.* Slaughtered animals, as well as those that have died because of disease, injury, or natural causes, are sources of meat, by-products, and rendered meals for pet food. Rendered products commonly found in dry pet food include chicken meal, poultry by-product meal, and meat and bone meal.

Animals that die on the farm may not be transported to the rendering plant for many days after death. These carcasses can be heavily contaminated with bacteria such as *salmonella* and *E. coli* released from the decomposing digestive tract. Dangerous *E. coli* bacteria are estimated to contaminate more than 50 percent of meat meals.

While the rendering process kills bacteria, it does not eliminate the endotoxins some bacteria produce during their growth. These toxins can survive processing, and can cause sickness and disease. Pet food manufacturers do not test their products for bacterial endotoxins.

In addition, flavorings such as "animal digest" that are sprayed onto dry food are commonly loaded with *Salmonella*, as numerous recalls and human illnesses have proven.

• *Drugs.* Because sick or dead animals are frequently processed for pet foods, the drugs that were used to treat or euthanize them may still be present in the end product. Penicillin and pentobarbital are just two examples of drugs that can pass through processing unchanged. Antibiotics used in livestock production also contribute to antibiotic resistance in humans.

• *Mycotoxins.* Toxins from mold or fungi are called mycotoxins. Modern farming practices, adverse weather conditions, and improper drying and storage of crops can contribute to mold growth. Pet food ingredients that are most likely to be contaminated with mycotoxins are grains such as wheat and corn; and fish meal. There have been many large pet food recalls in response to illness and death in pets due to a very powerful poison, called aflatoxin, in dry food.

- *Chemical Residues.* Pesticides and fertilizers may leave residue on plant products. Grains that are condemned for human consumption by the USDA due to residue may legally be used in pet food.

- *Acrylamide.* This carcinogenic compound forms at cooking temperatures of about 250°F in foods containing certain sugars and the amino acid asparagine (found in large amounts in potatoes and cereal grains). It forms during a chemical process called the Maillard reaction. Most dry pet foods contain cereal grains or starchy vegetables such as potatoes, and they are processed at high temperatures (200–300°F at high pressure during extrusion; baked foods are cooked at well over 500°F). These conditions are perfect for the Maillard reaction. In fact, the Maillard reaction is *desirable* in the production of pet food because it imparts a palatable taste, even though it reduces the bioavailability of some amino acids, including taurine and lysine. The amount and potential effects of acrylamide in pet foods are unknown.

7. **Preservatives:** Preservatives are not needed in canned foods since canning is itself a preserving procedure. Dry food manufacturers need to ensure that dry foods have a long shelf life (typically twelve to eighteen months).

Potentially cancer-causing agents such as BHA, BHT, and ethoxyquin are permitted at relatively low levels in pet and some human foods. The use of these chemicals in pet foods has not been thoroughly studied, and long term build-up of these agents may ultimately be harmful. Ethoxyquin has never been tested for safety in cats. Despite this, it is commonly used in well-known veterinary "prescription" diets.

8. Liver Disease: The liver is first in line to receive all the blood returning from the digestive tract. That's because the liver is a major detoxifying organ, with enzyme systems in place to intercept and dismantle many potential poisons. Large numbers of white blood cells also reside in the liver, ready to attack invading organisms.

The liver is also responsible for making many proteins, such as albumin; it makes cholesterol, the base molecule for important hormones; and it produces bile, which is essential for digestion and absorption of fats.

Cats' livers are particularly sensitive to dietary changes. If a cat does not eat, the liver gets stressed and starts calling for "reinforcements." In the cat's case, this consists of fat break-down around the body, which the liver then grabs from the blood stream and packs into its cells. This extreme fat hoarding can become so serious that it prevents cells from functioning properly, and a life-threatening type of liver failure, called "hepatic lipidosis" (fatty liver disease) can result. Overweight cats, and cats eating mostly or only dry food, are most at risk.

9. Allergies and Asthma: You may have heard that 80 percent of the immune system is found in the gut. While that isn't quite accurate, huge numbers of white blood cells do live in groups ("Peyer's Patches") along the intestinal lining. That makes sense, since the gut is one of the primary routes of entry into the body for invading organisms, from viruses to worms.

As mentioned briefly above, the high-heat processing that dry food undergoes during manufacturing can denature proteins, meaning that it distorts their shape. To a protein, shape is everything, and only a protein in the correct shape will function properly. Shape is also how the immune system identifies proteins that belong in the body ("self") versus foreign proteins. Viruses, bacteria, fungi, and other invaders are all identified by the proteins found on their surfaces. When an immune cell identifies a foreign protein, a whole cascade of signaling for reinforcements and production of antibodies is set into motion. Antibodies then scour the bloodstream looking for invaders matching their shape; when they find one, they latch on and signal for support. Inflammation is one of the primary responses.

When an abnormal protein is picked up by an immune cell and antibodies are produced, then every time that protein appears, antibodies flock to it and stimulate inflammation. More bad proteins, more inflammation.

The gut doesn't take kindly to this reaction, and will start rejecting the food—one way or another—vomiting or diarrhea. Cats seem to be especially good at (or perhaps fond of) vomiting, and indeed, vomiting is the primary symptom of food allergies, as well as full-blown inflammatory bowel disease.

A true food allergy is different from a dietary intolerance—though the symptoms may be the same. An allergy involves the immune system, while an intolerance may simply be a reaction to something in the food—one of the colorings, texturizers, or other additives. Allergies are generally to proteins; but there are proteins not only in meat, but also in corn, wheat, and other grains.

Both food allergies and dietary intolerances are more common with dry food. Fortunately, they both respond to dietary therapy.

10. Kidney and Bladder Stones: Both dogs and cats can develop inflammation, crystals, and stones in their bladders and kidneys. These conditions are exacerbated, if not outright caused, by dry food.

Cats get a condition called "feline lower urinary tract disorder" (commonly referred to as FLUTD, or sometimes by the older, outdated term, FUS—feline urologic syndrome) is not a single disease. In fact, it comes in at least three distinct varieties:

Cystitis—This term means "inflammation of the bladder." The majority of LUTD cases (about two-thirds) falls into the category of "idiopathic cystitis" (bladder inflammation of unknown cause). This syndrome in cats is very similar to interstitial cystitis in women. It is rare for bacteria to be involved—most are "sterile" inflammations.

Crystalluria—This is a condition where mineral crystals form in the bladder. There are many types of crystals in dogs, but only two are common in cats: struvite (also called magnesium-ammonium-phosphate), and calcium oxalate. Male cats who block usually have crystals that are held together in a matrix with mucus from the irritated bladder. This "plug" can slither down the urethra, where it can become stuck where the urethra narrows at its end.

Urolithiasis—A "lith" is a stone, and of course "uro" means it's in the urinary system. Only about 20 percent of LUTD cases involve bladder stones—about half of these are struvite, and half are calcium oxalate stones. They form most easily when the urine is very concentrated, which maximizes the chances of the components—which are all normally in urine—banging and sticking together into crystals or stones. Struvite stones can be dissolved by temporarily feeding an acidifed veterinary diet (the canned version, please!), but calcium oxalate stones must be removed surgically.

Dogs also get cystitis, crystals, and stones. However, in dogs, these conditions are more likely to be caused by bacteria, partly because so many dogs must hold their urine for many hours while their guardians are at work or school. The urinary system's natural defenses include urine flowing through out and washing bacteria along with it. When urine is held, bacteria have many hours to colonize the bladder and start causing havoc.

The best way to prevent all bladder problems is to keep lots of fluid flowing through the urinary system to flush these problem particles out. The dehydrating quality of dry food produces highly concentrated urine that is much more likely to form crystals and stones. Wet food is needed to keep the urinary tract healthy; and it's essential in any dog or cat with a history of bladder disease.

To give your pet the moisture and protein content that are so necessary for good health, try canned, homemade, or raw food.

Even though canned food is processed, it's cooked only once (briefly at lower heat), rather than twice at high heat for dry food (once when the animal products are rendered, and again during extrusion). Canned food also tends to have a much higher protein content than dry food.

Homemade food is ideal, if you are following a balanced recipe. (**Warning:** most "cookbooks" and recipes on the Internet are NOT balanced, and can cause serious harm over time.)

When you make your pet's food, you are 100 percent in control of the quality of the ingredients, and you can add additional supplements depending on your pet's individual needs, rather than getting a "one size fits all" commercial pet food.

Raw-meat-based diets can be made at home, or purchased frozen or freeze-dried. Even just adding a little raw meat to any commercial diet will be an improvement. However, raw meat is always contaminated with bacteria, and may even harbor worms and other parasites.

Dr. Hofve, many of our readers wish to know what pet foods they can buy from a store. This, as you know, is a complicated question. What pet foods do you suggest to your clients?

The most reputable manufacturers of "superpremium" and "natural" foods agree with holistic veterinarians that the very best diet for your animal companion is one that you make yourself. A homemade diet, carefully balanced nutritionally, and using raw and organic foods, is closest to what Mother Nature intended. However, many of us do not have the resources to make our pets' food, especially for multiple animals or large dogs. So, for those of us who rely, partially or entirely, on commercial foods for our animals, here are some guidelines to use in selecting a good-quality diet.[143]

Contents: The name of a pet food is strictly defined and tells us what is actually in the food.

- "Chicken Dog Food" must contain at least 95 percent chicken (excluding water).

- "Fish and Giblets for Cats" must be 95 percent fish and giblets together, and there must be more fish than giblets, since fish appears first on the label.
- If the label says "dinner," "platter," "entree," "nuggets," "formula," or similar term, there must be 25 percent of the named ingredients. That is, "Fish Dinner" must contain 25 percen fish.
- If more than one ingredient is named, such as "Fish and Giblets Entree," the two together must comprise 25 percent of the total, and the second ingredient must be at least 3 percent. A food labeled "Fish and Giblets Entree" may contain anywhere between 13 percent fish and 12 percent giblets, to 22 percent fish and 3 percent giblets.
- Ingredients labeled as "with" must be present at 3 percent, such as "Fish Dinner with Giblets."
- An ingredient labeled as a "flavor," such as "Beef Flavor Dinner," may not actually contain beef meat, but more likely will contain beef digest or other beef by-products that give the food a beef flavor.

That said, there are a couple of caveats that you should be aware of:

- It used to be that non-meat ingredients didn't count on the main label, so food labeled "Chicken and Rice Dinner" still had to contain 25 percent chicken. However, the rules have changed, so now "Chicken and Rice Dinner" could contain 13 percent chicken and 12 percent rice and be legally labeled.

- Multiple studies have found many mislabeled pet foods and treats. In some cases, ingredients are present in the food but not disclosed on the label; this is a serious problem if a pet has a food allergy, because the food may contain undeclared allergens. On the other hand, some products contained none of the primary ingredient as stated on the label. The pet food industry has thus far demonstrated no interest whatsoever in fixing the problem, although regulators are aware of it, and are looking for a solution.

When selecting a commercial food for your animal companion, be sure to read the label. Although percentages are misleading due to the variable moisture content of processed foods, they are often the only data available.

- Avoid foods containing "by-product meal," "meat and bone meal," or euphemisms like "beef and bone meal," which tend to be the least expensive (and thus poorest quality) animal-source ingredients. "Meat and bone meal" (MBM) is the mammal equivalent to "by-product meal" (which applies only to poultry). MBM was reported as the ingredient most likely to contain the drug used for euthanasia (sodium pentobarbital) in a study conducted by the FDA.
- A named meat or meat meal should be the primary protein source, rather than a cereal like corn gluten meal. Corn in all its forms must also be avoided.

The feed-grade corn used in pet food is certain to be genetically engineered. In low-priced foods, corn gluten meal is often substituted for expensive meat ingredients. Wheat is also a common allergen; wheat products should be avoided. All grains are susceptible to mold and other toxins.

- Never feed "semi-moist" type foods, which are full of additives, colorings, texturizers, and preservatives.

- Avoid foods containing chemical preservatives such as ethoxyquin, BHA, BHT, propylene glycol, or propyl gallate. Many brands are now preserved with Vitamins C and E instead of chemical preservatives. While synthetic preservatives may still be present, the amounts will be less.

- In general, select brands promoted to be "natural." While they are not perfect, they tend to be better than most.

- Stay away from "light" or "senior" or "special formula" foods. These foods may contain acidifying agents, excessive fiber, and inadequate fats that will result in skin and coat problems.

- Avoid generic or store brands; these may be repackaged rejects from the big manufactures, and certainly contain cheaper—and consequently poorer quality—ingredients.

- Change brands or flavors of dry food every two or three months to avoid deficiencies or excesses of ingredients, which may be problematic for your animal. Whenever you are changing foods, remember to GO SLOWLY. Add a tiny amount of new food to old, and gradually increase the proportion of new food. It will take a week or two to properly transition a cat.

- With canned food, you can change flavors daily if you wish—my cats prefer it that way!
- Cats need *at least 50 percent* of their diet (preferably 100 percent!) in the form of wet food (canned or homemade). Include a variety of meats and flavors to prevent finicky behavior and food allergies and intolerances. *Cats who are overweight, diabetic, or have a history of or current liver, pancreas, bladder or kidney disease, should not eat any dry or semi-moist food at all.*
- If you must feed dry food, remember to never get it wet. Do not mix with canned food, milk, broth, or water. All dry foods have bacterial contamination on the surface, and moisture will allow those bacteria to grow. Some are dangerous, and cause vomiting and/or diarrhea.

Above all, supplement with organic raw meats (meat should be frozen at -4°F for seventy-two hours, then thawed prior to use; follow safe meat-handling procedures at all times). If desired, a small amount lightly steamed, pureed or finely grated nonstarchy vegetables (they cannot be very well digested by carnivores otherwise). Dogs may be supplemented with tofu and cooked grains; however, cats should receive minimal carbohydrates in the diet. Be aware that plant products tend to raise urine pH and may contribute to bladder stones and urinary tract disease. Other helpful supplements include Omega-3 fatty acids, acidophilus, digestive enzymes, and Vitamins C and E.

For more information on Dr. Jean Hofve, her holistic pet care practice, books she has written on pet health, and for free access to a vast array of incredibly helpful articles on proper pet foods and health care, visit her website at www.LittleBigCat.com.

Conclusion

The Story Behind This Book[144]

By Joe Ardis, Dog Behavior Expert and
Certified Professional Trainer/Instructor

The world as we have created it is a process of our thinking.
It cannot be changed without changing our thinking.
—ALBERT EINSTEIN[145]

I haven't always cared about animals the way I do now. But then, something happened that changed the way I looked at everything: mankind, animals, God, and the world. Once I came to care, I knew this book had to be written.

This is my story. Bear with the sarcasm and humorous naïveté that befits my old self, because the ending is a story of redemption.

There was a time, not long ago in fact, that I wouldn't have even thought about what was going on in the pet food industry. Like many, I assumed some proverbial "they" were seeing to it that nothing harmful would make its way to a beloved animal's dish. And it wasn't just that I didn't *know*;

it's not a stretch to say that I wouldn't have made it a priority to do much about it had I known, simply because my relationship with even the word "pets" had been stunted. Sure, I *absolutely* cared about animal welfare from a distance, and I felt remorse and sadness when I heard of an animal being senselessly abused or killed. Any news regarding unnecessary harm to any of what I believe to be God's creation (including plant life) was stirring to me, merely because I was solid in my beliefs that as humans, we have a responsibility to look after the earth that God placed us upon as the dominating species. But beyond this, I had other things going on, and the creation of this planet would have to come second to the busyness of my all-consuming roles as a career man and father.

As a child, I grew up in a home that had very little experience with owning pets, and when our family did adopt a pet, it was with less-than-ideal commitment. If the animal didn't fit into our environment early on—which, in our house, meant that they had to be there for cuddling when you were in the mood, only bark at intruders, protect the humans of the residence, and remain obedient the rest of the time—they were rehomed. If they barked, chewed on stuff, got under your feet, or caused significant inconvenience, then they "just weren't working out," a conclusion that imprinted itself within my psyche from childhood forward into my adult life. Without ever analyzing that thought process to the point of fixing it, because animals were not a priority for me, I stagnated. I was seasoned in a slow-cooker that had propagated the same casual attitude toward animals that many have today, one that asserts that they are here for our pleasure only, and any inconvenience they bring is likely be a severance of that relationship if a quick fix cannot be implemented.

Needless to say, as a family, we never knew what we were doing when we brought an animal home. I look back and laugh at the methods of "correcting bad behavior" that we exercised in those days. We used silly time-outs at the wrong times, while orally lecturing the pets about elaborate plots related to undesirable behavior, assuming they would have any clue what it was we were carrying on about. By the time I was living on my own for the first time, I had arrived at a stifled outlook that would remain for several years, all but prohibiting me from ever committing to another pet animal. To say that it went as far as a "discomfort" around animals, despite how unintentional that mind frame had been implemented, would not be stretching the truth. Slowly I had become someone who was intimidated merely by the unwanted contact with a pet, even in someone else's home. Pets were, as my thinking had developed, largely inconvenient to humankind. Their hair, their noses, their tongues…all of it represented something "gross" that just *had* to be touched in order to connect with them. Then, I would reflect back now and again to my childhood and think, *Boy, I'd never do that again.* And what was the purpose of adopting (and touching) an animal? Companionship? I had led a life so close to my human family, the need to connect with an animal wasn't present. We had a mutual understanding, pets and I, that we didn't need each other.

Well, of course I owned an occasional, modest fish aquarium (its purpose in my home far more defined by the level of aesthetics it could bring to the ambiance of my living room than by the life of the fish within), but as far as the ever-faithful companion figure depicted in every nostalgic scene of the all-American dream home, I wasn't buying it.

When I looked at happy, Norman Rockwell-style paintings of young boys in overalls hugging the family dog in the grass next to their Radio Flyer wagons, my mind would wander to a scene wherein lies only a cacophony of noise-making furry things, muddy hairballs, and dripping, soggy tongues reaching their germs toward the unsuspecting humans from beyond their unbrushed teeth. When visiting the home of someone who chose willingly to coexist with these hairy "family members," my arms would involuntarily rise into the air well above wet-nose height while I continuously backed away from the animal until it could be ushered into a back room—all the while, my eyes darting about for a gallon of hand sanitizer in the case of accidental bodily contact.

I'll admit it: My discomfort with pets, primarily dogs, was not only overkill, it was often bordering on a clinical phobia as the result of my inexperience in regards to them—an inexperience I was perfectly content to hold onto for all my days.

But that was *before* a canine companion changed my life forever…

After relentless pleading over the period of several years from the three ladies in my life (my wife and two little girls), I could no longer ignore their requests (a convincing harmony of "please Honey," "please Daddy," and one "pwease Dai-dai" from my toddler); therefore, I caved in, allowing my soft heart to pave the way for the fifth member of our family. His name was "Tank" (a mastiff/boxer mix, because why not have a "tongue-on-legs" be useful as a guardian as well as companion, right?).

Oh sure, the first day was beautiful, sentimental, and endearing—the ultimate scene to trump any Rockwell painting, indeed: proud parents looking over the shoulders of their two pajama-donned, messy-haired, bright-eyed beauties on Christmas morning as they tore the colored paper from the box and held high the wiggling prize from within. I even caught myself thinking once or twice that the puppy was rather cute. *Yeah...Maybe I really could do this. Maybe I had it in me after all to be a dog owner...*

How could I have known that by allowing this innocent present-opening ritual in my own home to include *him*, I was really attending the coronation ceremony of the new king? By nightfall, it was revealed to me who really was master over whom, as I found I'd been demoted—reduced to naught but the dog-food vending machine: a slave in service to the seemingly eternal wants, whims, and requirements of the *new* master of the house. He was hungry; he was needy; he was clingy; he chewed on stuff; he barked; he required a trainload of attention and management; he pulled against the leash at three o'clock in the morning when he should have been going potty anywhere *but* that walkway!

Oh, the responsibility.

I honestly wondered at times if there would ever be normalcy in our home again; I wondered if we would be better off without him; I wondered if the tasks of puppy rearing would ever come to an end; I wondered the things a lot of people wonder when first committing to a family pet. And then, the day he issued a possessive warning growl toward my little girl over his bone, I wondered if he would ever turn on my wife or my daughters when I wasn't around.

That day presented me with a difficult choice. In the past, I would have been tempted to rehome this dog solely based on the enormous inconveniences to our lifestyle he presented, but I had gone into the arrangement this time with determination to see him be the American dream dog for our home. This time, it wasn't about me. It was about the wife and kids. After I observed his interaction with my daughter, however, my new-found determination was waning. I sat and stewed over the conundrum with confusion and doubt. Here I was, having finally done the unthinkable, opening my home to a pet with hair, a nose, and a tongue. For the sake of the family, I had embraced the duties that accompanied puppyhood, tackled all obstacles full steam ahead, and learned to grit my teeth until the reassuring, hand-to-fur contact of an animal was becoming gradually more tolerable to me. I was invested. I had even learned to...*care* about him.

But despite any progress or growth on my end in these areas, my lacking in knowledge of how to handle dog behavioral problems was suddenly glaringly apparent. It didn't work like it did in those lame Disney movies. You don't just bring home a dog, pat him on the head, toss a Frisbee, and crank out a productive and devoted family guardian who knows the difference between protecting his family from danger and protecting his bone from the family. The truth hit me like a freight train: I was going to have to get rid of the potential danger in my home, or learn to correct it—fast!

In a panic, I shared my woes with Eileen Pallotto, a friend from church who runs a local dog rescue mission and pet grooming shop. (Thank you, Eileen! It all started with you…) She quickly provided my wife and me with the contact information for an acquaintance of hers who came with her highest recommendation. Within days, my first session with Daren Pappas, a veteran dog behavior expert/trainer and certified pet technician (who has since become a dear friend over the years), took place, and within hours of that, I had taken my first step toward true enlightenment. Daren was filled with passion and enthusiasm for the care, treatment, and rehabilitation of animals, paralleled only by his passion and enthusiasm to share said knowledge.

I learned so many things so fast—tips and tricks the likes of which were far displaced from the average, failing methods I had casually observed from other pet owners and within my childhood home over the years. I learned that bursting into a room with your arms flailing around and voice at excited volumes when the dog is getting into something only serves to confuse a dog and invite him into your escalated chaos. I learned that shouting out the window at a barking dog in an effort to tell him to be quiet only communicates that you are happy to *join* him in his curious canine diatribe against the squirrel under the bush. I learned that attempting to retrieve an item from the dog's mouth via the grab-and-yank method only incites a fun game of tug-of-war. These techniques are about as effective as running around in a circle yelling, "Me too! Me too! Me too!"

Did you know that you cannot apply human psychology to an animal? Well, that was just absurd…

My understanding of basic dog behaviors was deficient the day I agreed to bring in our companion. Right away, it was clear that my own understanding of dog behavior could not be trusted, as they were greatly shaped from a lifetime of incorrect animal/human relationship concepts. It was the revealing of this dysfunction in my own nature that exposed the deepest need to abandon all that I had ever known (or thought I knew) about animals, dogs or otherwise, in trade for a *radical* change in my worldview.

Little by little, by applying the things I had learned from Daren, small goals were met on a daily basis. We all felt it: an ongoing restoration of law and order within the home. I started recognizing a change in my dog. Yes, *my* dog. He was becoming so much more than something I merely tolerated; he was becoming a friend. Like they talk about in the movies and on TV about a dog being "man's best friend," I found myself actually enjoying his company and respecting him as his own entity with individual quirks and characteristics. In getting to know Tank, I started to truly love him as I observed the traits of his protective and affectionate personality with my family.

By opening my heart to something dramatically new and harnessing each opportunity to learn all that God would teach me in uncharted territory, I began to see God's design, and His real intention for people coexisting with animals. My stress and anxiety in relation to animals and mankind's bond with them was a result of my own weak, human nature and my unwillingness to venture out of the realm of what was familiar and secure. The more I welcomed the lessons in front of me, the more those lessons began to bleed into other areas of my life until my perspectives on many things around me had been given a complete overhaul. If an animal—one that I might have nervously avoided at a friend's house and never thought of again—could become one of the most valued treasures within my existence (just outside of family and close friends), then perhaps I had missed out on other enjoyable areas of life because of shallow impressions.

I began to see what an incomplete person I had been as a whole. I discovered that there were interests I never knew I had, expressions of life and art and music and emotion that had been disregarded by the hasty dismissals of my youth. I expanded my mind: movies I had written off because they appeared from the cover artwork that they weren't my style were now proving themselves to be some of the best stories I had ever seen; music I had shrugged off because the beat reflected a demographic I didn't feel I had fit into, I now found myself grooving to; foods I had refused to taste because they were too bizarre by description or picture were quickly replacing my favorite dishes; others' artistic expressions through dance that I had thought were "boring" now revealed the level of dedication, talent, and persistence they demanded to be well-executed (and that alone was reason enough to appreciate them); comedy that I thought had been too trivial or off-beat soon became outrageously funny; moments I would have allowed my children to ignore new experiences were now becoming an opportunity to help them expand *their own* minds and try new things; unfamiliar methods that God might be able to use in peoples' life were showing their true usefulness beyond my typical cavalier perceptions.

It was suddenly so obvious to me that I had never been challenged to grow beyond myself—that I had been content to exist within the perimeters of periphery prejudice, embracing things that fit me, and discarding things that didn't match the box-worldview I had constructed. As a result, it *also* became suddenly obvious that I wasn't connecting to other people with the sincerity God had intended me to… All this because of a dog.

However, unexpectedly, as I became closer to my clever and ever-growing tail-wagger, a profound truth halted me in my tracks.

I didn't change Tank. He changed me.

None of this was ever about my skills as a dog handler. God was training me, and using Tank to do it.

Simply becoming a healthy and concerned pet parent was not enough. This experience birthed a passion within me to help others who were showing the same limited approach to animals I had once exhibited, assisting them with the psychological or emotional hang-ups related to a more professional behavioral problem resolution. Without hesitation, I enrolled in a certification program, my sights set on becoming a dog trainer. Little did I know that would only be the beginning.

Early on in these new endeavors, I came upon "Sealey," an adorable Pomeranian with a troubled past.

Sealey had been bred in a puppy mill. Her life was confined to a cage. Her sole human interaction was moments when she would be lifted by the scruff of her neck and carelessly tossed into a breeding pen between her heat cycles. The conditions she had been living in were horrendous and deplorable. A dear friend of the family and master animal trainer, Jenny Keist, is a devoted woman who has spent her love and everything she owns to being the "sanctuary," her own personal animal rescue, having extended her love and patience to an uncountable number of animals (of all various species), and who was involved in busting and shutting down the puppy-mill where Sealey had been kept. Sealey's first loving connection to humankind and initial steps toward rehabilitation were through Jenny. Yet Jenny, whose home was filled to the brim already with animals requiring her attention and care, could not keep her. I stepped in and agreed to foster Sealey temporarily.

Sealey had *major* behavioral issues. She didn't trust humans (understandably), and showed extreme dominance around children or people with higher energy levels. She habitually faced a complete shutdown whenever she was exposed to large groups of people as a lack of proper socialization. The handling of her leash brought new demands on her existence, and her hindquarters were not to be touched. I had small children, so this lovely little dog, as neglected as she had been and as much as I wanted to care for her, was never going to be prioritized above my own family. I limited her contact with those in my home while I actively sought to rehome her, but finding a new family for a fearful and aggressive dog is difficult if not impossible in some areas (we live in a modest community largely considered to be a retirement area), so I knew that rehabilitation was needed in order to make that happen. I had no way of knowing whether or not I would be the human who would make a breakthrough, but I at least had to try.

Tank had been a puppy when we got him, so my connection with him required the patience of one molding a blank canvas into something beneficial and wholesome from the start. Sealey was a new experience. Her canvas had been spotted and torn by those who had hurt her, and the only means to rehabilitation would be through slowly and patiently mending the damage done by others.

As I began to work with her, I almost immediately spotted a glimmer of sweetness beneath her hardened exterior. Somewhere under all those growls, nips, shutdowns, freak-out sessions, and constant jumpiness was a very loving dog, and my determination to appeal to that part of her started to grow. The encounter to foster her became longer than I had originally expected, and it certainly was not without its challenges. Every time she began to open up and show visual signs of trust and confidence toward new people and situations, her initial response would result in a temporary relapse into her old countenance, and I would have to extend further patience and effort to bring resolve.

Some days I was searching high and low for a new home for her, all the while, other days, I would observe her with guarded affection, wondering if maybe…just *maybe*…we might be her family.

Over time, she began to participate in loving interaction with those she had previously been intimidated by, and her aggression diminished. Gone were the days I had to stand between her and my children. The leash and hindquarters had become nonissues. Days turned into weeks, weeks became months, and before I knew it, we had cared for her a whole year. She wasn't even comparable to the dog we had committed to rehoming as a favor to Jenny. Through expanding my horizons to work with a troubled animal, God had, *once again*, shown me another aspect of His intended connection between humans and animals. Not just "connection"…but reconciliation. Redemption. Expansion of what both humans and animals *can* be, when allowed to grow beyond the box they have constructed.

After many trials and successes, Sealey was given a permanent home. She lives with us to this day.

As the course of my trek through canine interaction played out, I reclaimed my rightful place as master of the house with Sealey, as Tank had long since become a pleasant family dog. And yes, as a family, we are now living within a healthy and pleasant balance at home, which consists of a father, a mother, now three little girls, a well-behaved guard dog, and an adorable, obedient, affectionate Pomeranian.

Today, I am a dog behavior expert, a certified professional trainer/instructor, and a registered professional therapeutic animal companion handler. I work with therapeutic animal organizations to bring happiness in hospice care and lend a hand to select animal rescue channels. I am the lead K-9 trainer at Whispering Ponies Ranch, a retreat facility devoted to ministering to those with special emotional needs, and I teach clinics at pet centers to dog owners looking to overcome issues such as canine dominance, fear, aggression, and other behavioral problems. And now, not only is Sealey a loving, obedient, and attentive pet, the rehabilitation process I presented her with has delivered this once socially handicapped, fearful, little doll into the role of a professional registered therapeutic companion dog. And believe me, she *adores* all of the attention she receives from the people she comforts.

Left here, this would be, on its own, a wonderful ending; would it not?

Yet, by learning how to communicate with one of God's amazing creations, and in the way *He* designed, I began to care about the needs of my pets as individuals. Tank and Sealey didn't choose to be adopted by our family, and they, like all other foster/therapy animals that have passed through our home, have had no choice regarding the food that they are given at each meal. They cannot speak in words we humans can understand when the food we give them makes them sick.

Immediately, my approach to pet parenting took a shift toward ensuring that my own pets not only lived happily, but thrived in their environment. A quick online search turned up uncountable red flags within the pet food industry. Having never heard of such things as "rendering plants," I was shocked and disgusted when related images and articles appeared on my screen, telling stories of euthanized or diseased animals being recycled into the very dish I feed them from. Having no previous knowledge of the dangers of preservatives and dyes and their adverse affects on animals, I was shocked to see the never-ending list of health-related trauma that ensues when a casual pet owner buys the poorest brands of food.

There was no way "they" would allow this to happen. Right?

But when I did a little further digging on who "they" really were, and the regulation holes that exist within the industry, I realized that change had to happen at home. My pets would never be fed these horrible foods. And, as you readers are now more aware, the journey from the poorest foods to the healthier foods presented a major problem. Since so many companies participate in the big commercial lie, and since corners will be cut everywhere they are allowed to be for the sake of money-mongers, it would not be as easy as running to the market to find a new brand. Terms I was at the time unfamiliar with, such as "by-product" and "Red 40," were everywhere, and information regarding the steps one can take to avoid them was scarce.

I began to fill my home library with books and materials discussing canine and feline food and health care. (Because I am allergic to cats, I do not personally own one, but I care deeply about them. Because several of my closest friends, clients, and colleagues own cats, my determination to educate myself on existing dangers extended to their species, also.) I had every intention of telling every person I knew about the things I was learning, the shocking and unbelievable practices happening right under all our noses, within the disguise of fancy packaging. The more I educated those I came into contact with, the more I realized that the general public was also completely unaware. How could this be such a serious problem that almost everyone knew nothing about?

Slowly, over time, my education of industry practice paved the way for me to raise awareness through social media outlets, television, radio, and written publications (many of those to whom I have reached out, like Shane and his dog Cookie mentioned earlier, have since changed their pet-feeding habits). I was driven by a passion to alert any and all who would hear me of the hazards of commercial pet foods. As I continued to learn, that passion spilled into pet medicine as well.

And just as I had felt the joy that resulted from the initial commitment I developed for Tank and Sealey, I began to experience a joy each and every time someone committed to providing a healthier life for their own beloved animal. Each step made by mankind toward the goal of comfortable cats and dogs was an achievement I could celebrate. I take great pleasure in seeing the quality of life for an animal and their handler/owner improve through further knowledge.

In early 2014, I approached Tom Horn of Defender Publishing with some of these pet food industry facts. He, too, was largely unaware of these issues, and immediately proposed that we work together to raise awareness through his media channels. Shortly after that initial conversation, fellow pet owner, researcher, best-selling author, and successful ghostwriter Donna Howell came on board to help me place what I had been learning into words. This book is the result.

If even one reader takes the initiative to provide a healthier living standard for his or her pet as a consequence of this book, all the work that went into it will have been worth it.

Afterword

By Sharon K. Gilbert,
author of *The Armageddon Strain*,
biologist, and mom to the
cutest dachshund in Missouri

In the sixty plus years since I was a little "pup," I've named and cared for half a dozen cats (who tended to run away, or so my farm parents told me), a canary, four hamsters, a few odd fish (aren't all fish odd?), a guinea pig, a calf, and more than two dozen tail-wagging dogs. This being said, you won't be surprised to hear that I love animals, which is why I'm writing this afterword. In truth, this book shocked me, and I pray that it shocked you as well, because our precious dogs, cats, hamsters, and iguanas deserve much better than we human "parents" have been giving them. God charged humans with dominion over animals, and that means that we love and protect them. I admit that I've failed at that charge, but that is about to change.

Can you say the same? If the information here has convicted you, then rejoice. Now is not the time for self-pity and regret, but for taking that conviction and beginning anew with your precious pup, parakeet, or piranha (and to those who nodded and said, "Gee, I wonder how she knew about my piranha tank," I say, "Why?"). Take stock of your pantry, your fridge, your medicine cabinet, and your life. Teach your children how to take loving dominion by becoming the best, truest friend his or her pet ever had.

And, once you've accomplished that, buy a few more copies of this book to give as gifts. The pooches of your neighborhood will thank you, and so will their humans.

Many thanks to Joe Ardis and Donna Howell for all their painstaking research and time spent writing. I can tell you from personal experience that both of these wonderful people are intelligent, incredible, talented, tenacious, and stalwart humans who have a deep affection for and affinity with animals of all kinds. My dachshund, Sam T., who staked a claim on my heart seven years ago, will no doubt give them a bucket load of thanks and kisses next time he sees them.

Now, put down this book and go hug your pet!

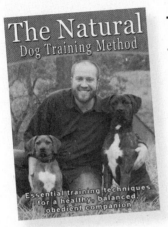

The Natural Dog Training Method

Join dog behavior expert, Joe Ardis, as he uniquely and innovatively approaches canine training from the dog's perspective.

The decision to bring a dog into your home can represent enormous and unexpected responsibility and chaos. Many of us find ourselves feeling overwhelmed when the reality of such a large undertaking is exposed and the market for training books and other information is so vast and competitive.

Effective techniques are taught in a concise and comprehensive manner, and apply equally to both the new dog owner and to those who are merely seeking to sharpen their pets' current behavior skills. Achieving optimum behavior from your dog requires understanding more than a memorized set of verbal commands, baby talk, or an elaborate training plot, which can lead to frustration and discouragement, and can prohibit progress. Joe Ardis relays in simple, easy-to-follow terms how understanding the thought patterns and psychological nature of your dog is essential to successful human/canine communication.

Chapters on this two-hour DVD include:

1. Sit
2. Stay
3. Down
4. The Correctional Touch
5. The Walk
6. Feeding by Invitation
7. Properly Giving Treats and Rewards
8. Claiming Spaces
9. Creating Areas
10. Affection by Invitation
11. Nipping
12. Crate Training
13. Housebreaking
14. Nutrition
15. Grooming and Maintenance

To learn more about proper pet care and to see some helpful training products, visit Joe Ardis' website, at www.HealthyPetGuru.com.

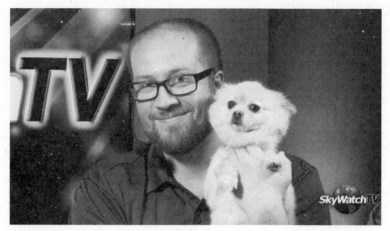

Joe Ardis with his registered professional therapy dog Sealey, as they make a special appearance on the popular television program, SkyWatch TV, to discuss the many benefits of therapeutic animal companionship!

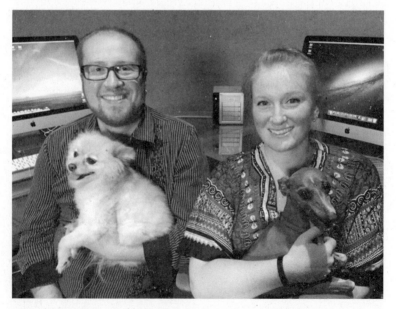

Joe Ardis with Sealey and Donna Howell with Zero.

Notes

1. Abraham Lincoln, "Abraham Lincoln > Quotes," *goodreads*, last accessed September 10, 2014, http://www.goodreads.com/quotes/9194-i-care-not-for-a-man-s-religion-whose-dog-and.
2. "U.S. Pet Ownership & Demographics Sourcebook (2012)," *American Veterinary Medical Association*, last accessed June 18, 2015, https://www.avma.org/KB/Resources/Statistics/Pages/Market-research-statistics-US-Pet-Ownership-Demographics-Sourcebook.aspx.
3. Gian Carlo Menotti, as quoted by *BrainyQuote*, last accessed October 10, 2014, http://www.brainyquote.com/quotes/quotes/g/giancarlom115993.html.
4. Adolf Hitler, "Adolf Hitler > Quotes," *goodreads*, last accessed October 17, 2014, http://www.goodreads.com/quotes/553-if-you-tell-a-big-enough-lie-and-tell-it.
5. "Pets by the Numbers," *Humane Society*, January 30, 2014, last accessed October 20, 2014, http://www.humanesociety.org/issues/pet_overpopulation/facts/pet_ownership_statistics.html.
6. "Americans Spent a Record $56 Billion on Pets Last Year," *CBS News Money Watch*, March 13, 2014, last accessed October 20, 2014, http://www.cbsnews.com/news/americans-spent-a-record-56-billion-on-pets-last-year/.
7. Ibid., emphasis added.
8. "Busting the Sugar-Hyperactivity Myth," *WebMD*, 1999, last accessed October 20, 2014, http://www.webmd.com/parenting/features/busting-sugar-hyperactivity-myth; emphasis added.
9. Therese J. Borchard, "Why Sugar Is Dangerous to Depression," *PsychCentral*, last accessed October 20, 2014, http://psychcentral.com/blog/archives/2011/07/13/why-sugar-is-dangerous-to-depression/.

10. "Anthony Reddick Sentenced for Deaths of 13 Pit Bulls," *Huffington Post*, last accessed June 16, 2015, http://www.mirror.co.uk/news/world-news/dog-fighting-thug-jailed-causing-4306068.

11. "Pet Food," *FDA U.S. Food and Drug Administration*, under the heading "FDA Regulation of Pet Food," last accessed November 17, 2014, http://www.fda.gov/AnimalVeterinary/Products/AnimalFoodFeeds/PetFood/default.htm#PetFoodContamination.

12. Marion Nestle, *Pet Food Politics: The Chihuahua in the Coal Mine* (University of California Press, Kindle Edition, 2008), Kindle locations 1818–1822.

13. "Get the Facts! Raw Pet Food Diets can be Dangerous to You and Your Pet," *FDA U.S. Food and Drug Administration*, last accessed November 17, 2014, http://www.fda.gov/AnimalVeterinary/ResourcesforYou/AnimalHealthLiteracy/ucm373757.htm.

14. Susan Thixton, "Is It an FDA Lie or FDA Neglect?" November 6, 2013, *Truth About Pet Food*, last accessed November 17, 2014, http://truthaboutpetfood.com/is-it-an-fda-lie-or-fda-neglect/.

15. "Is it Really FDA Approved?" *FDA U.S. Food and Drug Administration*, under the heading "FDA Regulation of Pet Food," last accessed November 18, 2014, http://www.fda.gov/ForConsumers/ConsumerUpdates/ucm047470.htm.

16. "Pet Food," *FDA*, emphasis added, http://www.fda.gov/AnimalVeterinary/Products/AnimalFoodFeeds/PetFood/default.htm#PetFoodContamination.

17. "FDA's Regulation of Pet Food," *FDA U.S. Food and Drug Administration*, last accessed November 18, 2014, http://www.fda.gov/AnimalVeterinary/ResourcesforYou/ucm047111.htm.

18. Ibid., emphasis added.

19. Ibid., emphasis added.

20. This insight was given by Allie Anderson in a personal phone call with author Donna Howell on November 20, 2014.

21. "Tea Trea Oil, *WebMD*, last accessed November 20, 2014, http://www.webmd.com/vitamins-supplements/ingredientmono-113-

tea20tree20oil.aspx?activeingredientid=113&activeingredientna me=tea20tree20oil.

22. Adrienne Weeks, "Tea Tree Oil Side Effects in Infants," last updated August 16, 2013, last accessed November 20, 2014, http://www.livestrong.com/ article/110517-tea-tree-oil-side-effects/.

23. "Inspections, Compliance, Enforcement, and Criminal Investigations: Ad-Med Biotechnology, LLC 8/12/14," *FDA U.S. Food and Drug Administration*, last accessed November 20, 2014, http://www.fda.gov/iceci/enforcementactions/ warningletters/2014/ucm410476.htm.

24. "Tea Tree Oil (Melaleuca Alternifolia)—Topic Overview," *WebMD*, last accessed November 20, 2014, http://www.webmd. com/skin-problems-and-treatments/tc/tea-tree-oil-melaleuca- alternifolia-topic-overview, emphasis added.

25. "FDA's Regulation of Pet Food," *FDA*, http://www.fda.gov/ AnimalVeterinary/ResourcesforYou/ucm047111.htm.

26. Ibid.

27. Ibid.

28. Ibid., emphasis added.

29. Ann N. Martin, *Food Pets Die For: Shocking Facts about Pet Food*, third ed. (New Sage Press, Troutdale, Oregon: 2008), 50.

30. AAFCO main home website, last accessed November 20, 2014, http://www.aafco.org/.

31. Ibid.

32. "The Business of Pet Food," *AAFCO*, under the heading "Did you know?" last accessed February 19, 2015, http://petfood. aafco.org/Home.aspx, all emphasis in original.

33. "Pet Food Labeling Requirements," *Pet Food Institute*, last accessed February 19, 2015, http://www.petfoodinstitute. org/?page=Labeling.

34. "About PFI," *Pet Food Institute*, last accessed February 19, 2015, http://www.petfoodinstitute.org/?page=About_PFI.

35. "AFRPS: Animal Feed Regulatory Program Standards," Introduction, *FDA*, launched January of 2015, last accessed February 23, 2015, http://www.fda.gov/downloads/ForFederalStateandLocalOfficials/AnimalFeedRegulatoryProgramStandardsAFRPS/UCM402506.pdf.

36. Ibid., emphasis added.

37. Ibid., emphasis added.

38. Martin, *Food Pets Die For*, 65.

39. Ibid.

40. Kurt Vonnegut, "Quotes about Health," *goodreads*, last accessed June 18, 2015, http://www.goodreads.com/quotes/tag/health.

41. "Rendered Products in Pet Food," *Dogs Naturally: The Magazine for Dogs without Boundaries*, last accessed March 30, 2015, http://www.dogsnaturallymagazine.com/rendered-products-in-pet-food/.

42. "Regulatory Information," *FDA U.S. Food and Drug Administration*, Section 201 (f), last accessed June 18, 2015, http://www.fda.gov/regulatoryinformation/legislation/federalfooddrugandcosmeticactfdcact/fdcactchaptersiandiishorttitleanddefinitions/ucm086297.htm; emphasis added.

43. "§342. Adulterated Food," section (a), *FDA U.S. Food and Drug Administration*, article in the U.S. Government Printing Office archives, last accessed June 18, 2015, http://www.gpo.gov/fdsys/pkg/USCODE-2010-title21/html/USCODE-2010-title21-chap9-subchapIV-sec342.htm.

44. Please note that the time signatures in this area refer mostly to the second half of one full-hour episode. The first half of the episode focused on unrelated material, so many citations are within the second half of the hour. Also note that time signatures refer specifically to the episode as it appears on Amazon Instant Video, http://www.amazon.com/gp/product/B007V6ZIU8/ref=dv_dp_ep1.

45. Host, Mike Rowe, produced by Pilgrim Films & Television, *Dirty Jobs*, episode entitled "Animal Rendering" (episode 14 in season 4 as it originally aired; episode 1 in season 4 as listed on Amazon Instant Video; episode 102 in the total series), *Discovery Channel*, first aired January 20, 2009, 1:22–1:32.

46. Ibid., 24:42–24:45.

47. Ibid., 25:40–25:57.

48. Ibid., 26:01–26:15.

49. Ibid., 26:39–26:57; emphasis added.

50. Ibid.

51. Ibid., 27:33–27:57; emphasis added where emphasis was spoken in the original.

52. Ibid., 30:17–30:24.

53. Ibid., 30:47–30:54.

54. Ibid., 31:15–31:26.

55. Ibid., 33:02–33:12.

56. Ibid., 33:19–33:27.

57. Ibid., 34:26–34:47.

58. Ibid., 35:03–35:14.

59. Ibid., 35:15–35:30.

60. Ibid., 36:15–36:25.

61. Original interview with Hersh Pendell, Kaiser, Oregon, news interview, 2000, viewable online here: "Former AAFCO President Admits Pet Food May Contain Pets," YouTube video, 0:18–0:43, posted by WeeMiniMoose, uploaded August 3, 2008, last accessed April 1, 2015, https://www.youtube.com/watch?v=RuoSxSJ94RY, emphasis placed where emphasis was spoken in the original.

62. Keith Woods, "The Dark Side of Recycling," *Earth Island Journal* (Fall 1990), emphasis added. A portion of this original article is viewable here: "The Shocking Truth about Commercial Dog Food," *Dog Food Advisor*, last accessed April 1, 2015, http://www.dogfoodadvisor.com/dog-food-industry-exposed/shocking-truth-about-dog-food/. PLEASE NOTE THAT THIS ARTICLE AT

THE CITED URL SHOWS DISTURBING IMAGES OF
ANIMALS IN A GRINDER; READER'S DISCRETION
ADVISED.

63. Dr. Wendell Belfield, DVM, "Food Not Fit for a Pet," *Let's Live Magazine* (May 1992). Full article viewable here: Dr. Wendell Belfield, DVM, "Food Not Fit for a Pet," *Frog Holler's Fila Brasileiro*, last accessed April 1, 2015, http://www.angelfire.com/biz/froghollerfilas/FoodBelfield.html; emphasis added.

64. "Pet Overpopulation," *Humane Society*, last accessed June 3, 2015, http://www.humanesociety.org/issues/pet_overpopulation/.

65. "NYC Veterinarian Charged with Dumping 35 Euthanized Cats, Dogs, and Lizard Alongside Highway, *The Associated Press*, last accessed June 3, 2015, http://news.yahoo.com/nyc-veterinarian-charged-dumping-35-euthanized-cats-dogs-191402939.html.

66. "What's REALLY in Your Pet's FOOD??" YouTube video, posted by slibby62, uploaded July 21, 2008, last accessed June 8, 2015, https://www.youtube.com/watch?v=g9DTzDfYMxo.

67. "Rendering Investigation," video embedded, *Last Chance for Animals*, last accessed June 8, 2015, http://www.lcanimal.org/index.php/investigations/investigations-in-the-field/rendering.

68. "Rendering Investigation," YouTube video, posted by Last Chance for Animals, uploaded May 15, 2009, last accessed June 8, 2015, https://www.youtube.com/watch?v=Wf0Eqxf5lD4.

69. Michael J. Sorba, "Firm Gives Remains of Euthanized Pets Another Use," February 8, 2010, *Contra Costa Times News*, last accessed June 8, 2015, http://www.contracostatimes.com/california/ci_14359793.

70. "Options for Animal Disposal," *Office of the County Veterinarian*, last accessed June 8, 2015, http://www.sandiegocounty.gov/reusable_components/images/awm/Docs/vet_disposaloptions.pdf.

71. This interview was conducted over an online messaging system on July 16, 2015, between Joe Ardis and Jenny Lynn.

72. "Food and Drug Administration/Center for Veterinary Medicine Report on the Risk from Pentobarbital in Dog Food," *FDA U.S.*

Food and Drug Administration, last accessed June 3, 2015, http://www.fda.gov/AboutFDA/CentersOffices/OfficeofFoods/CVM/CVMFOIAElectronicReadingRoom/ucm129131.htm.

73. Ann Martin, *Food Pets Die For*, 34–35.

74. "FAQs," *Animal Cancer Foundation*, last accessed June 3, 2015, http://www.acfoundation.org/faq/faq.php.

75. "The Recycling of Our Pets," YouTube video, 0:52–1:03, posted by Jonny Kahleyn-Dieb, uploaded February 10, 2009, last accessed June 9, 2015, https://www.youtube.com/watch?v=0QylPWG_d0k.

76. Ibid., 1:09–2:03.

77. "The Shocking Truth about Commercial Dog Food," *Dog Food Advisor*, last accessed June 9, 2015, http://www.dogfoodadvisor.com/dog-food-industry-exposed/shocking-truth-about-dog-food/.

78. "A Graphic Description of What the FDA Allows in Pet Food," *Truth about Pet Food*, October 31, 2009, last accessed June 9, 2015, http://truthaboutpetfood.com/a-graphic-description-of-what-the-fda-allows-in-pet-food/.

79. Stephanie Simon, "Outcry over Pets in Pet Food," *LA Times*, January 6, 2002, last accessed June 9, 2015, http://articles.latimes.com/2002/jan/06/news/mn-20784.

80. Lynn Stratton, "Find Out What Is Really in Your Pet's Food," *Healthy Holistic Living*, last accessed June 9, 2015, http://www.healthy-holistic-living.com/rendered-pet-food.html.

81. "Regulatory Information," *FDA*, Section 201 (f), last accessed June 18, 2015, http://www.fda.gov/regulatoryinformation/legislation/federalfooddrugandcosmeticactfdcact/fdcactchaptersiandiishorttitleanddefinitions/ucm086297.htm; emphasis added.

82. "§342. Adulterated Food," section (a), *FDA U.S. Food and Drug Administration*, article in the U.S. Government Printing Office archives, last accessed June 18, 2015, http://www.gpo.gov/fdsys/pkg/USCODE-2010-title21/html/USCODE-2010-title21-chap9-subchapIV-sec342.htm.

83. "CPG Section 675.400 Rendered Animal Feed Ingredients,"
    FDA U.S. Food and Drug Administration, last accessed June
    18, 2015, http://www.fda.gov/ICECI/ComplianceManuals/
    CompliancePolicyGuidanceManual/UCM074717; emphasis
    added.
84. "CPG Section 690.500 Uncooked Meat for Animal Food,"
    FDA U.S. Food and Drug Administration, last accessed June
    18, 2015, http://www.fda.gov/ICECI/ComplianceManuals/
    CompliancePolicyGuidanceManual/ucm074712.htm; emphasis
    added.
85. Ibid.
86. "Grains? In Commercial Pet Food?" *The Whole Dog*, last accessed
    June 22, 2015, http://www.thewholedog.org/id52.html.
87. Ryan Jaslow, "Journal Retracts Genetically Modified
    Corn Study that Found Tumor Risks in Rats,"
    November 29, 2013, *CBS News*, last accessed
    June 11, 2015, http://www.cbsnews.com/news/
    journal-retracts-genetically-modified-corn-tumor-rats-study/.
88. Cheryl Lock, "What Is GMO Food for Pets?" *Pet 360*, last
    accessed June 15, 2015, http://www.pet360.com/dog/nutrition/
    what-is-gmo-food-for-pets/2LlW3Iwrik2MvegksbvNvg?intcid=L
    INKART.
89. Brandy Arnold, "The Dangers of Genetically Modified
    Ingredients in Dog Food," *The Dogington Post*, April 6, 2015,
    last accessed June 15, 2015, http://www.dogingtonpost.com/
    the-dangers-of-genetically-modified-ingredients-in-dog-food/.
90. Thomas and Nita Horn, *Forbidden Gates: How Genetics, Robotics,
    Artificial Intelligence, Synthetic Biology, Nanotechnology, and
    Human Enhancement Herald the Dawn of Techno-Dimensional
    Spiritual Warfare* (Defender Publishing, Crane, MO: 2010),
    155–157.
91. "Study on Genetically Modified Corn, Herbicide, and Tumors
    Reignites Controversy," *CBS News*, last accessed June 11, 2015,
    http://www.cbsnews.com/news/study-on-genetically-modified-
    corn-herbicide-and-tumors-reignites-controversy/.

92. "What is GMO?: Agricultural Crops that Have a Risk of Being GMO," *Non-GMO Project*, last accessed June 11, 2015, http://www.nongmoproject.org/learn-more/what-is-gmo/.

93. "GMO FACTS: Frequently Answered Questions," *Non-GMO Project*, last accessed June 11, 2015, http://www.nongmoproject.org/learn-more/.

94. "FDA's Role in Regulating Safety of GE Foods," *FDA U.S. Food and Drug Administration*, under the heading "Labeling," last accessed June 11, 2015, http://www.fda.gov/forconsumers/consumerupdates/ucm352067.htm; emphasis added.

95. "What is GMO?" *Non-GMO Project*, http://www.nongmoproject.org/learn-more/what-is-gmo/

96. "Ethanol Poisoning in Dogs," *Pet MD*, last accessed June 15, 2015, http://www.petmd.com/dog/conditions/neurological/c_dg_ethanol_toxicosis.

97. Linda Bonvie, "High Fructose Corn Syrup Turns Up in the Oddest of Places," *Food Identity Theft*, July 5, 2012, last accessed June 15, 2015, http://foodidentitytheft.com/high-fructose-corn-syrup-turns-up-in-the-oddest-of-places/.

98. "Ingredients to Avoid," *The Dog Food Project*, last accessed June 15, 2015, http://www.dogfoodproject.com/?page=badingredients.

99. "Food Quality and Wholesomeness," *Dog Cat Home Prepared Diet*, last accessed June 15, http://dogcathomeprepareddiet.com/Food%20Quality%20and%20Wholesomeness.html.

100. Jodi Ziskin, "Why Many Pet Foods Contain MSG and Why You May Not Even Know It," *Holistic Healthy Pets*, last accessed June 15, 2015, http://holistichealthypets.net/2012/10/05/why-many-pet-foods-contain-msg-and-why-you-may-not-even-know-it/.

101. Ibid., emphasis added.

102. Linda P. Case, *Canine and Feline Nutrition: A Resource for Companion Animal Professionals* (Mosby: 1995), 93.

103. Mark Morris, Mark Lone and Hand, Michael Lewis, *Small Animal Clinical Nutrition III* (Mark Morris Associates: 1990), 1–11.

104. "Do Dogs and Cats Need Grains?" *Natural Pet Productions*, last accessed June 22, 2015, http://www.naturalpetproductions.net/articles/npp.grains.pdf.

105. I. H. Burger, *The Waltham Book of Companion Animal Nutrition* (Pergamon: 1995), 10; 26–27.

106. T. J. Dunn, DVM, "Contrasting Grain-Based and Meat-Based Diets for Dogs," *Pet MD*, last accessed June 22, 2015, http://www.petmd.com/dog/nutrition/evr_dg_contrasting_grain_based_and_meat_based_diets.

107. Dr. Jean Hovfe, Holistic Veterinarian, "Top 10 Myths about Pet Food and Nutrition," *Only Natural Pet*, last accessed June 22, 2015, http://www.onlynaturalpet.com/holistic-healthcare-library/food-diet---general/147/top-10-myths-about-pet-food-and-nutrition.aspx.

108. Dr. Ken Tudor, "Grain Free—Is It Really the Answer?" *Pet MD*, last accessed June 22, 2015, http://www.petmd.com/blogs/thedailyvet/ktudor/2012/august/is_grain_free_really_the_answer-26668.

109. "Grains? In Commercial Pet Food?" http://www.thewholedog.org/id52.html.

110. Ibid.

111. "Grains Are Very, Very Bad for Your Obligate Carnivore Cat, Carnivore Dog," *Best Cat and Dog Nutrition*, last accessed June 22, 2015, http://www.bestcatanddognutrition.com/roger-biduk/grains-are-very-very-bad-for-your-carnivore-cat-carnivore-dog/.

112. "Grains? In Commercial Pet Food?" http://www.thewholedog.org/id52.html.

113. "Canine Diseases Linked to Grains in Dog Food (Part 1)," *Dog Food Advisor*, last accessed June 22, 2015, http://www.dogfoodadvisor.com/dog-food-industry-exposed/grains-in-dog-food-1/.

114. "Entomological Notes," *College of Agricultural Sciences, Penn State University*, last accessed June 22, 2015, http://ento.psu.edu/extension/factsheets/pdf/flourgrainmite.pdf.
115. L. G. Arlian et al, "Serum immunoglobulin E against storage mites in dogs with atopic dermatitis," *American Journal of Veterinary Research*, January 2003, 32–36; 64, http://www.ncbi.nlm.nih.gov/pubmed/12518875.
116. J. W. Bennett and M. Klich, "Mycotoxins," *US National Library of Medicine*, July 16, 2003, last accessed June 22, 2015, http://www.ncbi.nlm.nih.gov/pmc/articles/PMC164220/; emphasis added.
117. "Aflatoxin Toxicosis: Get the Facts," *Oregon Veterinary Medical Association*, last accessed June 22, 2015, https://oregonvma.org/care-health/aflatoxin-toxicosis-get-facts.
118. The research for this section of the book was conducted considering the following sources, not necessarily in this order. All online material last accessed June 23, 2015. If specific book pages are available, those instances are individually cited: "Ingredients to Avoid," *The Dog Food Project*, http://www.dogfoodproject.com/?page=badingredients; related searches on the FDA official website, *U.S. Food and Drug Administration*, http://www.fda.gov/; "Pet Food Ingredients Revealed," *Natural News*, last accessed June 23, 2015, http://www.naturalnews.com/Report_pet_food_ingredients_8.html; "These Pet Food Preservatives Could Be Toxic to Your Pet," *Dog Food Advisor*, http://www.dogfoodadvisor.com/red-flag-ingredients/dog-food-preservatives/; "5 Ingredients You NEVER Want to Find in Your Dog's Food," *I Love Dogs Online*, http://iheartdogs.com/5-ingredients-you-never-want-to-find-in-your-dogs-food/; "Preservatives in Dog Food—The Good and the Bad," *SlimDoggy*, http://slimdoggy.com/preservatives-in-dog-food-the-good-and-the-bad/; "Pet Food Ingredients A to Z," *Petnet*, http://www.petnet.io/pet_health_blogs/pet-food-ingredients-a-to-z-ascorbic-acid#.VYh65vlVikp; Linley Dixon, PhD, "Is Your Pet's Food as Safe as You Think?" *The Cornucopia Institute*,

December 9, 2014, http://www.cornucopia.org/2014/12/pets-food-safe-think/?gclid=CNO_-d6RpsYCFQguaQodS9wBlQ; "Artificial Food Dyes and Pet Food," *Well Minded Pets*, http://www.wellmindedpets.com/blog/2013/11/25/the-dangers-of-artificial-dyes-in-pet-food; "EWG's Dirty Dozen Guide to Food Additives: Generally Recognized as Safe—But Is It?" *EWG*, November 12, 2014, http://www.ewg.org/research/ewg-s-dirty-dozen-guide-food-additives/generally-recognized-as-safe-but-is-it?gclid=CK-ek4yVpsYCFQ-raQodrLoFYQ#butylated-hydroxyanisole; Dominique De Vito, *Green Dog, Good Dog* (Lark Books, New York, London: 2009); Richard H. Pitcairn, DVM, PhD, and Susan Hubble Pitcairn, *Dr. Pitcairn's Complete Guide to Natural Health for Dogs & Cats* (Rodale: 2005, third ed.).

119. Benjamin Franklin, "Benjamin Franklin > Quotes," *goodreads*, last accessed July 7, 2015, http://www.goodreads.com/quotes/247269-an-ounce-of-prevention-is-worth-a-pound-of-cure.

120. "The Biggest Myths about Raw Food (and Why They're Mostly Nonsense)," *Healthy Pets*, April 8, 2013, last accessed June 25, 2015, http://healthypets.mercola.com/sites/healthypets/archive/2013/04/08/raw-food-diet-part-2.aspx.

121. "Floor Sweepings and Other Shameful Dog Food Ingredients—Oh My!" *Dog Food Advisor*, last accessed June 30, 2015, http://www.dogfoodadvisor.com/choosing-dog-food/dog-food-grain-by-products/.

122. "Tocopherols," *Organic Technologies*, last accessed June 30, 2015, http://www.organictech.com/FoodNutritionalIngredients/Tocopherols.aspx.

123. "Purina Sues Blue Buffalo for False Advertising and Disparagement," *Pet Food Honesty*, last accessed July 7, 2015, http://www.petfoodhonesty.com/pressrelease.php.

124. Ibid.

125. Ibid.

126. "Blue Buffalo Admits to [Lying to] Consumers, Lawsuit with Purina Heats Up," *Poisoned Pets*, last accessed July 7, 2015, http://www.poisonedpets.com/blue-buffalo-admits-to-bullshitting-consumers/.

127. Ibid.

128. "Purina Sues Blue Buffalo," *Pet Food Honesty*, http://www.petfoodhonesty.com/pressrelease.php.

129. Daniella Silva, "Lawsuit Claims Purina's Beneful is Poisoning, Killing Dogs," February 24, 2015, *NBC News*, last accessed July 7, 2015, http://www.nbcnews.com/news/us-news/lawsuit-claims-purinas-beneful-poisoning-killing-dogs-n312176.

130. Jodi and Lisa Hernandez, "Dogs Were 'Poisoned': Discovery Bay Man Sues Purina after His Dogs Die, Get Sick," February 26, 2015, *NBC News*, last accessed July 7, 2015, http://www.nbcbayarea.com/news/local/Dogs-Were-Poisoned-Discovery-Bay-Man-Sues-Purina-After-His-Dogs-Die-Get-Sick-294255971.html.

131. Dr. Jean Hofve, "Selecting a Good Commercial Pet Food," *Little Big Cat*, last accessed July 13, 2015, http://www.littlebigcat.com/nutrition/selecting-a-good-commercial-pet-food/.

132. Paracelsus, "Paracelsus Quotes," *Brainy Quote*, last accessed July 9, 2015, http://www.brainyquote.com/quotes/quotes/p/paracelsus170321.html.

133. For more information on this ingredient, read the following assessment reports: "Imidacloprid—Human Health and Ecological Risk Assessment—Final Report," *USDA Forest Service*, last accessed July 8, 2015, http://www.fs.fed.us/foresthealth/pesticide/pdfs/122805_Imidacloprid.pdf; "IMIDACLOPRID: SAFETY SUMMARY for VETERINARY Use on Dogs and Cats. Poisoning, Intoxication, Overdose, Antidote," *PARASITIPEDIA*, last accessed July 8, 2015, http://parasitipedia.net/index.php?option=com_content&view=article&id=2688&Itemid=2995.

134. For more information on this ingredient, read the following: "Pyrethrin and Permethrin Toxicity in Dogs and Cats," *Pet Education*, last accessed July 8, 2015, http://www.peteducation.com/article.cfm?c=2+1677&aid=2252.

135. For more information on this ingredient, read the following: "Amitraz Toxicity in Dogs and Cats," *Pet Education*, last accessed July 8, 2015, http://www.peteducation.com/article.cfm?c=2+1677&aid=2230.

136. "Is Cedar Safe for Cats?" *Wondercide*, last accessed July 9, 2015, http://www.wondercide.com/is-cedar-safe-for-cats/.

137. "Rose Geranium Oil," *Web MD*, last accessed July 8, 2015, http://www.webmd.com/vitamins-supplements/ingredientmono-153-rose%20geranium%20oil.aspx?activeingredientid=153&activeingredientname=rose%20geranium%20oil.

138. Dr. Karen Becker, "How Much Money Are You Wasting On Pet Vaccines?" March 10, 2010, *Healthy Pets*, last accessed July 9, 2015, http://healthypets.mercola.com/sites/healthypets/archive/2010/03/31/high-cost-of-pet-vaccinations.aspx.

139. Dr. Karen Becker, "Dog and Cat Vaccines Are NOT Harmless Preventative Medicine," August 20, 2012, *Healthy Pets*, last accessed July 9, 2015, http://healthypets.mercola.com/sites/healthypets/archive/2012/08/20/pets-over-vaccination-disease.aspx.

140. "Holistic Pet Vaccinations," *HolVet: Holistic Veterinary Services*, July 9, 2015, http://www.holvet.net/pet_vaccinations.html.

141. As quoted in a personal phone call between Donna Howell and Dr. Jean Hofve, June, 2015.

142. Note that much of this information was derived from Dr. Jean Hofve's article "10 Reasons Why Dry Food Is Bad for Cats & Dogs," *Little Big Cat*, last accessed July 13, 2015, http://www.littlebigcat.com/nutrition/why-dry-food-is-bad-for-cats-and-dogs/. Used with permission.

143. Note that much of this information was derived from Dr. Jean Hofve's article "Selecting a Good Commercial Pet Food," *Little Big Cat*, last accessed July 13, 2015, http://www.littlebigcat.

com/nutrition/selecting-a-good-commercial-pet-food/. Used with permission.

144. A portion of this conclusion has been taken from the following source: Thomas Horn, Terry James, Joe Ardis, et al, *Do Our Pets Go to Heaven?* (Defender Publishing, Crane, MO: 2013), foreword. However, please note that the original material included here was written and copyrighted by Joe Ardis. No copyright infringement has occurred by this subsequent use of said material.

145. Albert Einstein, "Albert Einstein> Quotes," *goodreads*, last accessed July 13, 2015, http://www.brainyquote.com/quotes/quotes/p/paracelsus170321.html.